Philip M. Hanno· David R. Staskin ·
Robert J. Krane· Alan J. Wein (Eds.)

Interstitial Cystitis

With 52 Figures

Springer-Verlag
London Berlin Heidelberg New York
Paris Tokyo Hong Kong

Philip M. Hanno, MD
Professor and Chairman, Department of Urology, Temple University
School of Medicine, Broad and Tioga Street, Philadelphia,
Pennsylvania 19140, USA

David R. Staskin, MD
Assistant Professor of Urology, Harvard Medical School, 330
Brookline Avenue, Boston, Massachusetts 02215, USA

Robert J. Krane, MD
Professor and Chairman, Department of Urology, Boston University
School of Medicine, 720 Harrison Avenue, Boston, Massachusetts
02118, USA

Alan J. Wein, MD
Professor and Chairman, Division of Urology, University of
Pennsylvania School of Medicine, 3400 Spruce Street, Philadelphia,
Pennsylvania 19104, USA

Front cover: Fig. 19.2. Rupture of bladder mucosa and submucosa at increased bladder distension.

ISBN 3-540-19598-X Springer-Verlag Berlin Heidelberg New York
ISBN 0-387-19598-X Springer-Verlage Berlin Heidelberg New York

British Library Cataloguing in Publication Data
Hanno. Philip M. *1948–*
    Interstitial cystitis
    1. Man. Bladder. Cystitis I.. Title 616.623
ISBN 3-540-19598-X

Library of Congress Cataloging-in-Publication Data
Interstitial cystitis/P. M. Hanno . . . [et al.], eds
p. cm.
ISBN 0-387-19598-X (alk. paper)
1. Interstitial cystitis. I. Hanno, Philip M.
[DNLM: 1. Cystitis. WJ 500 1616] RC921. C9157 1990 616.6' 23—dc20
DNLM/DLC
for Library of Congress   90-9568
                                                              CIP

Typeset by MJS Publications, Buntingford. Printed by Henry Ling, Dorchester.
2128/3916-543210 Printed on acid-free paper

Preface

Until recently interstitial cystitis was considered a urologic curiosity, a rare problem with relatively specific diagnostic criteria that many urologists would see only once or twice in a decade. This has changed drastically in the last ten years. Interstitial cystitis is now a very controversial subject that has ignited the interest of physicians in general, urologists in particular, basic scientists and even government agencies. It is a potentially much more common and more devastating disorder (or group of disorders) than had been believed. The exponential growth in clinical and basic research is largely due to the efforts of patient groups who demanded that more attention be paid to this problem. We owe them a debt of gratitude for putting interstitial cystitis in the spotlight and quite literally under the microscope.

In this book we have attempted to put together the current views of experts from around the world regarding the many aspects of this disorder. It is hoped that we can provide an image of where we stand as we enter the 1990s. If the book can stimulate other physicians and basic scientists to enter this exciting field of research, and if it can provide hope to the many thousands of patients who suffer from this disease, we will consider it a success.

Acknowledgement

This book is dedicated to the Interstitial Cystitis Association and its hundreds of members who have contributed so much of their time and effort toward making this disease less of a mystery.

We would also like to thank our wives. Their patience during the many months spent on preparation of the manuscript is gratefully acknowledged.

January 1990

Philip Hanno
David Staskin
Robert Krane
Alan Wein

Contents

5 Interstitial Cystitis: Animal Models
M.R. Ruggieri, F.C. Monson, R.M. Levin, A.J. Wein and

6 Etiology: Etiologic and Pathogenic Theories in Interstitial Cystitis
M. Holm-Bentzen, J. Nordling and T. Hald 63

Editorial Comment
Etiologic Theories: Deficiency of the Bladder Lining
D.R. Staskin

SECTION 3 DIAGNOSIS

7 Light Microscopic Findings in Bladders of Patients with Interstitial Cystitis
S.L. Johansson

Contributors

F. Aldenborg
Assistant Professor, Department of Pathology, University of
Göteborg, Göteborg, Sweden

K.E. Andersson
Professor of Pharmacology, Department of Clinical Pharmacology,
University Hospital, Lund, Sweden

G.S. Benson
Professor of Surgery, Department of Urology, University of Texas
School of Medicine, Texas Medical Center, Houston, Texas, USA

M.A. Cann
Research Associate, The Urban Institute, 2100 Main Street NW,
Washington, DC, USA

L. Enerbäck
Professor of Pathology, University of Göteborg, Göteborg, Sweden

M. Fall
Associate Professor of Urology, Department of Urology, Sahlgren's
Hospital, University of Göteborg, Göteborg, Sweden

B. Fransden
Department of Clinical Chemistry, Kolding Hospital, Kolding,
Denmark

T. Hald
Chief Urologist, Herlev Hospital, Copenhagen, Denmark

P.M. Hanno
Professor and Chairman, Department of Urology, Temple University
School of Medicine, Philadelphia, Pennsylvania, USA

P.J. Held
Senior Research Associate, The Urban Institute, 2100 Main Street
NW, Washington, DC, USA

H. Hedlund
Department of Urology, University Hospital, Lund, Sweden

M. Holm-Bentzen
Research Associate in Urology, Department of Urology, Herlev
Hospital, Copenhagen, Denmark

A. Ingelman-Sundberg
Chairman, Department of Obstetrics and Gynecology, Karolinska
Institute, Stockholm, Sweden

S.L. Johansson
Professor, Department of Pathology and Microbiology, University of
Nebraska Medical Center, Omaha, Nebraska, USA

R.M. Levin
Research Professor of Pharmacology in Urology, University of
Pennsylvania School of Medicine, Philadelphia, Pennsylvania, USA

G. Lose
Department of Urology, Rigshospitalet, University of Copenhagen,
Denmark

T. Malloy
Clinical Professor of Urology, University of Pennsylvania School of
Medicine, Philadelphia, Pennsylvania, USA

J. Mattila
Department of Pathology, Tampere University Central Hospital,
Tampere, Finland

E. McGuire
Professor and Chairman, Department of Urology, University of
Michigan Hospital, Taubman Center, Ann Arbor, Michigan, USA

F.C. Monson
Research Assistant Professor of Pharmacology in Urology,
University of Pennsylvania School of Medicine, Philadelphia,
Pennsylvania, USA

A. Nehra
Urodynamics Fellow, Department of Urology, Boston University
School of Medicine, Boston, Massachusetts, USA

J. Nordling
Chief Urologist, Herlev Hospital, University of Copenhagen,
Denmark

K.J. Oravisto
Former Head of the Urological Division, University Central
Hospital, Helsinki, Finland

M.V. Pauly
Professor of Economics and Health Care Systems, University of
Pennsylvania, Philadelphia, Pennsylvania, USA

C. Lowell Parsons
Associate Professor of Surgery and Urology, School of Medicine,
University of California Medical Center, San Diego, California, USA

S. Raz
Professor of Urology, UCLA Medical School Center for Health
Sciences, Los Angeles, California, USA

M.R. Ruggieri
Research Assistant Professor, Division of Urology, University of
Pennsylvania, Graduate Hospital, Philadelphia, Pennsylvania, USA

G. Sant
Associate Professor, Department of Urology, Tufts University
School of Medicine, Boston, Massachusetts, USA

A. Shanberg
Clinical Professor of Surgery and Urology, University of California at
Irvine, Los Angeles, California, USA

A. Siegel
Department of Urology, Hackensack Medical Center, Hackensack,
New Jersey, USA

D.R. Staskin
Assistant Professor of Urology, Harvard Medical School, Boston,
Massachusetts, USA

A.R. Stone
Assistant Professor, Department of Urology, School of Medicine,
University of California at Davis, Sacramento, California, USA

Y. Vardi
Department of Urology, Rambam Medical Center, Haifa, Israel

A. Walsh
President, Société Internationale d'Urologie, 4 Donnybrook Close,
Dublin 4, Eire

G. Webster
Associate Professor of Urology, Duke University Medical Center,
Durham, North Carolina, USA

A.J. Wein
Professor and Chairman, Division of Urology, University of
Pennsylvania, Philadelphia, Pennsylvania, USA

K.E. Whitmore
Graduate Hospital, Philadelphia, Pennsylvania, USA

Section 1

Introduction

Chapter 1

Interstitial Cystitis: An Introduction to the Problem

A.J. Wein, P.M. Hanno and J.Y. Gillenwater

Even for those of us who are experienced at saying a lot about a little, it is difficult to write an introductory chapter about a condition for which few specific diagnostic criteria have been established and for which there is no agreed pathophysiology, evaluation, or treatment. "Interstitial cystitis" (IC) is a term that is applied in different ways by different people to describe a constellation of symptoms and sometimes signs that some people group under the overall heading of "sensory disorders of the bladder and urethra", while others prefer to use the inclusive term "the painful bladder" or "painful bladder syndrome" (PBS). When we were residents, interstitial cystitis implied a small capacity fibrotic bladder which had resulted from a panmural inflammation of unknown etiology. Once tuberculosis and carcinoma in situ had been ruled out, there was little to do except contemplate an augmentation cystoplasty for symptom relief. No one gave much thought to how the bladder got that way once the important "rule outs" were excluded, and no one gave much thought to whether there was a population of patients with a more moderate or milder form of the condition. Subsequently, it became obvious that there was a large number of adult patients, predominantly women, with a chronic, painful, and variably incapacitating disorder of the urinary bladder, a small percentage of whom developed this "end stage" bladder picture, but the rest of whom did not and who continued to complain bitterly of symptoms, albeit with some remissions and exacerbations, for which physician after physician had no logical explanation. In the United States, it was the efforts of such frustrated patients, and especially Dr. Vicki Ratner, then an orthopedic resident in New York City, which led to the formation of the Interstitial Cystitis Association (ICA). Within this group, it became readily apparent that common complaints included unsympathetic physicians, inordinate delays in diagnosis, and frequent misdiagnoses of a psychosomatic disorder in an anxious, neurotic, or psychoneurotic patient. The ICA was originally organized to educate patients and to serve as a support group, and has become an educational group, not only for patients, but for physicians who are unfamiliar with the disease. Largely through the educational efforts of the ICA, and through their very successful lobbying activities with Congress, more and more attention came to be focused upon IC. An initial interstitial cystitis working group was formed by Dr. Ratner and Drs. Gary Striker and Charles Rodgers of the National Institutes of Health in 1986, and a workshop, sponsored by the National Institute of Arthritis, Diabetes, Digestive and Kidney Diseases (NIDDK) was organized and held in August of 1987. The goals of the workshop, which might also serve as goals for any volume on IC, were outlined as follows:

1. Provide a framework for acceptance of exact criteria on which to base a diagnosis of IC. What is it and who has it?

2. Better define the patient population with IC and work towards establishing a national registry. Who has it, how many people have it, and what are the epidemiologic characteristics of the group? Is there anything to be learned about the disease from its epidemiologic characteristics?

3. Determine the state of science in each of the areas concerned with IC. Interdigitate more closely basic and clinical science efforts in the study of IC. Do our assumptions, "folklore", and methods of evaluation and treatment make any scientific sense? Is there any consensus on how to diagnose the disease, and is there any sense of what a proper algorithm for diagnosis and treatment should include?

4. Establish definitive areas ready for research initiatives in IC. Where do we go from here?

Although the goals were certainly touched upon, it was apparent, after two and a half days discussion, that there were many opinions by respected and intelligent people from not only the clinical sciences but also the basic sciences, but that there was little consensus about any specific issue, except in the most general of terms. The workshop has been recently summarized in the *Journal of Urology* (140:203–206, July 1988), and the content of the summary provides a useful pot-pourri of the relevant issues. We gratefully acknowledge the publishers, Williams and Wilkins Co., and the Editor of the *Journal of Urology*, who have graciously given permission to reproduce this workshop summary in its originally published form as a part of this introductory chapter. The summary, with its references, follows.

SUMMARY OF THE NATIONAL INSTITUTE OF ARTHRITIS, DIABETES, DIGESTIVE AND KIDNEY DISEASES WORKSHOPS ON INTERSTITIAL CYSTITIS, NATIONAL INSTITUTES OF HEALTH, BETHESDA, MARYLAND, 28–29 AUGUST, 1987 AND 22 NOVEMBER, 1988

Interstitial cystitis is a syndrome characterized by urinary frequency nocturia, urgency, suprapubic pressure and pain with bladder filling, many times relieved by emptying. Urine cultures and cytology studies are negative. There is no precise definition for interstitial cystitis. The etiology and pathogenesis of the disease are unknown.

Bourque introduced the concept of painful bladder disease, which includes any combination of unexplained frequency, urgency, dysuria, incontinence, suprapubic or perineal pressure or pain, discomfort, hesitancy, weak stream, feeling of incomplete emptying, malaise and dyspareunia.[1] Conditions included in painful bladder disease would be the urethral syndrome, interstitial cystitis and prostatosis.

In 1915 Hunner reported on 8 women with a history of suprapubic pain, frequency, nocturia and urgency lasting an average of 17 years.[2] Cystoscopically, he described the presence of either ulcers or linear cracks in these patients. Hunner's ulcer actually is seen only rarely in these patients.[3] Walsh first described mucosal glomerulations as "red strawberry-like dots that often coalesce to become hemorrhagic spots which ooze blood from the bladder mucosa on second filling of the bladder under anethesia". This has become one of the important diagnostic criteria of interstitial cystitis.[4]

Drs. Philip Held, Philip M. Hanno, Alan J. Wein and Mark Pauly presented the data from their recent epidemiological study of interstitial cystitis. The survey was derived from questionnaires involving several groups, including board certified urologists, the last patient diagnosed by each of these urologists, the last patient treated by each of these urologists, and a group of patients from the Interstitial Cystitis Association and a group from the general population. Doctor Held reported that there are 20,000 to 90,000 diagnosed cases of interstitial cystitis in the United States, the upper boundary estimate for undiagnosed interstitial cystitis is about 4 to 5 times that number, the minimum benefit of cure is based on an estimate of 44,000 patients (which amounts to 428 million dollars per year) and the quality of life of women with interstitial cystitis was substantially below that of white women with end stage renal disease. In a previous epidemiological study in Finland Oravisto estimated the prevalence as 18.1 female patients per 100,000 female population.[5] He estimated an annual incidence of 1.2 new female patients per 100,000 per year. Thus, the prevalence in the United States was twice that found by Oravisto. In the Held study the median age of onset was 40 to 50 years, with a duration of 7 to 10 years. The average interval from onset to diagnosis was 30 to 50 months.

Five studies were presented in the Pathology-Pathophysiology section. Drs. Sonny L. Johansson, Claes Anderstrom and Magnus Fall described the morphological changes in the bladders of patients with interstitial cystitis. The findings are based on 25 patients with nonulcerative disease, 43 with classical (ulcer) disease, and controls with reflux and stress incontinence. Doctor Johansson does not believe that early nonulcerative cases progress to the classical ulcerative disease. In the classical disease an ulcer was found in 100 per cent of the cases, granulation tissue in 98 per cent, mucosal hemorrhage in 85 per cent, intense mononuclear infiltrate in 91 per cent and perineural inflammatory infiltrate in 71 per cent. In the nonulcerative form of the disease relatively unaltered mucosa was seen in 88 per cent of the cases with some mucosal rupture in 94 per cent and suburothelial hemorrhage in 72 per cent. Scanning electron microscopy showed that the interstitial cystitis patients had less surface mucin than normal control patients.

Dr. Douglas Harrington, and Doctors Fall and Johansson described the immunohistochemical and cytofluorometric analyses of the bladder mucosa in the aforementioned patients. In the early disease there was some T-cell infiltrate but in the classical disease there were more intense T-cell infiltrates with B-cell nodules. It is not known if this is a specific immunological response in interstitial cystitis or a nonspecific manner of responding to noxious stimuli.

Dr. Liennart Enerback discussed the role of mucosal mast cells in interstitial cystitis. There are 2 distinct mast cell populations observed in interstitial cystitis, 1 in the mucosa and 1 in the muscle layer. The mucosal mast cells are formaldehyde-sensitive while those in the muscle layer are not. In ulcerative (classical) interstitial cystitis the mucosal mast cells are increased only in the area of the ulcer. In the early form of the disease no increased mucosal mast cells are seen. Mast cells were increased in the muscle layer in the interstitial cystitis patients but more so in those with ulcers.[6]

Dr. David Lagunoff presented a pathological perspective on the pathogenesis of interstitial cystitis. Interstitial cystitis is an inflammatory disease and the mediators, such as leukotrienes, kinins or platelet aggregating factors, have not been identified. The disease is localized to the bladder but why this is so is not known. Is it owing to something in the urine or because of immunological targeting? Also, it is a chronic disease clinically and pathologically, showing mononuclear cell infiltrate. Finally, some cases progress with fibrosis.

The third session dealt with neuropharmacology and neurophysiology of the bladder. Dr. William D. Steers described the afferent innervation of the bladder. Hypogastric and pelvic nerves contain the afferents. The neuropeptide transmitters for the afferents include substance P, vasoactive intestinal polypeptide, calcitonin gene-related peptide, peptide histidine isoleucine, Galanin and L-enkephalin. Substance P could be the mediator for the inflammatory response. It causes vasodilation, increases vascular permeability, degranulates mast cells of histamine, causes bladder contraction and promotes polymorphonuclear leukocyte migration. Capsaicin is a substance that causes release of neurotransmitters from small unmyelinated C afferent fibers. Chronic administration depresses the micturition reflex, abolishing micturition in the neonate but not in adult animals. As far as afferents and pain are concerned there is a specificity theory (individual stimuli and fibers for pain, temperature and distension). Another theory is that 1 fiber may do everything but the type of sensory appreciation may simply vary with the intensity of the stimulus.

Dr. Edward J. McGuire discussed the pathophysiology of hypersensitive bladders and postulated that hypersensitivity most likely has a different neurological pathway than does reflex activity. The hypersensitive bladder indicates a subjective sensation of a need to void. The sensation of having to urinate must be a nonspecific symptom, since patients with the bladder drained by a catheter have a desire to void despite an empty bladder. With motor urge incontinence urine passage often is the first sensation. With anticholinergics capacity may increase but if an involuntary contraction is going to occur the warning time may not change. Through this type of argument and others Doctor McGuire concluded that cortical sensation may, indeed, be subserved by another pathway than reflex activity.

Doctor Wein discussed mechanisms of drug action on the lower urinary tract and stated that most drugs available affect the muscle contractile activity rather than the hypersensitivity states. He noted that propantheline is almost exclusively an atropine-like agent, while oxybutynin, dicyclomine and flavoxate are musculotropic relaxants (antispasmodics) with varying atropine-like properties. Other substances acting on the bladder are prostaglandin inhibitors, calcium antagonists, β-adrenergic agonists, tricyclic antidepressants (particularly imipramine), antihistamines, mucosal anesthetics, phenazopyridine hydro-chloride, dimethylsulfoxide (intravesical), oxychlorosene (intravesical) and heparin, and other glycosaminoglycan analogues.

The pharmacology of the lower urinary tract was described briefly but, again, this has been evaluated mostly from the standpoint of the motor side and in terms of receptors that are either agonists or antagonists for bladder smooth muscle contraction. Cholinergic excitatory receptors exist throughout the bladder smooth muscle and these doubtless account for at least the main portion of the emptying contraction seen with pelvic nerve stimulation. The concept of atropine resistance was discussed and references that argue against the presence of atropine resistance in normal men likewise were listed. Atropine resistance provides a tempting explanation for the lack of total efficacy of the anti-muscarinic agents in the patients with detrusor hyperactivity. The problem is that interstitial cystitis and other disorders concerned with the painful bladder and urethra generally are not associated with evidence of bladder hyperactivity, either phasic involuntary bladder contractions or tonic decreased compliance. To better understand these disorders pathways and receptors that subserve the sensory side of bladder activity as well as what various stimuli actually do in the normal and diseased bladder must be better understood. For instance the implication of this ties in well with other talks that mentioned the arachidonic acid cascade and the liberation of substances through the cyclooxygenase and lipoxygenase pathways, which might be mediators of pain and inflammation. Just as we do fairly well in disorders of hyperactivity with drugs designed specifically to inhibit bladder activity, so might we do as well in patients with hypersensitivity – with drugs designed to inhibit one or another phase of the sensory side of response to stimuli.

In section 4 Drs. Walter E. Stamm, Anthony J. Schaeffer and Edward M. Messing discussed whether interstitial cystitis is an infectious disease. There is no evidence that interstitial cystitis is caused by aerobic or anaerobic bacteria, viruses, Chlamydia, Ureaplasma, Mycobacterium hominis, herpes simplex virus, cytomegalovirus and adenovirus. Doctor Messing also spoke on the role of noninfectious inflammatory diseases in interstitial cystitis. Evidence for this concept included the epidemiological findings and lack of other etiologies, positive and negative histopathological findings, anti-bladder antibodies found in some studies, possible relationships to allergic phenomenon, the response of some patients to anti-inflammatory medications, and presence of eosinophils and mast cells. Evidence against this concept of a noninfectious inflammatory disease includes not much inflammation present, the finding of antibladder antibodies (soft data), titers of antinuclear antibodies not high and no relationship of the titers to the course of the disease. Other evidence against an infectious etiology are the lack of predictable response to anti-inflammatory agents and the fact that urinary diversion gives total relief even though the bladder is still there. There is no evidence that urethritis or vaginitis can lead to interstitial cystitis. Doctor Messing says that many patients with bacterial cystitis have bladder mucosal glomerulations when the bladder is distended. There is no evidence that a neuropathic virus is causing the bladder hypersensitivity.

In section 5 Dr. Harold Carron discussed pain and neuroanatomy and how they relate to interstitial cystitis. Doctor Carron noted that the definition of the chronic pain syndrome fits interstitial cystitis. He believes that frequency and urgency probably are mediated through the parasympathetic nervous system primarily and the distension symptoms probably are mediated through the sympathetic nervous system primarily. He described unmyelinated and finely myelinated fibers on the sensory side but he noted that there were no specific pain fibers for interstitial cystitis. Doctor Carron discussed the gate control theory of pain and small unmyelinated fibers stimulating the action system while large unmyelinated fibers inhibited the action system. He also spoke about the descending antinociceptive tracts in the spinal cord. He noted that in pain clinics what we see is the pain behavior. However, the sequence is nociception to pain to suffering to pain behavior. We do not see the suffering and this really is an important part of the chronic pain syndrome. Acute pain is distinguished from chronic pain. Acute pain includes pain as a symptom that is biologically useful and associated with anxiety. Narcotics are useful and there is little addiction potential. A pathological condition is recognized, and cure and relief are likely. In chronic pain pain is the disease. There is no biological usefulness to the pain and it is associated with depression. Narcotics are contraindicated and patients often are polyaddicted. There is a complex interaction between physical and psychological aspects, and cure or relief may not be possible. Factors influencing chronic pain behavior include implication of injury and probability of outcome, past experience, ethnic and cultural influences, secondary gain possibility and psychological make-up. Characteristics of chronic pain include alteration in life style (no pleasurable activities), failure of progressive improvement, suffering inappropriate to the evident somatic problem, multiple intractable complaints, depression, anxiety, neurotic behavior, no realistic future plans, excess analgesic use, history of multiple operations, circadian rhythm disturbance, unresponsiveness to treatment and pre-morbid characteristic of passive dependency.

Drug abuse in the chronic pain syndrome occurs with benzodiazepines (60 per cent), codeine (50 per cent), oxycodone (50 per cent) and opiates (25 per cent). Treatment for the chronic pain syndrome includes electrical stimulation, which is effective in sympathetic disorders and probably works at least somewhat by increasing blood flow. It is interesting that patients who smoke do not respond well to electrical stimulation. Electrical stimulation has to be done only 2 to 3 times a day and the effects will last for 24 hours. Tricyclic antidepressants are used in patients with pain but they are not used as antidepressants. These compounds block pain arousal. It should be noted that the tricyclic antidepressants also were mentioned in the discussion of treatment of the hyperactive bladder and the role of amitriptyline (or potential role) in interstitial cystitis patients also was mentioned. It is used by some people to treat the symptoms of interstitial cystitis and the mechanism of action most likely is not that of an antidepressant. Doctor Carron believes that tricyclic antidepressants block pain arousal and that doxepin might be the most effective in this regard, while amitriptyline is the second most effective. He notes that imipramine does not have as good a result in pain as doxepin or amitriptyline. He also discussed the anticonvulsants, including phenytoin, carbamazepine and valproic acid. It was useful to add valproic acid to a regimen of amitriptyline. Valproic acid acted somewhat like baclofen in that it inhibited the reuptake of gamma aminobutyric acid, an inhibitory neurotransmitter in the spinal cord. Doctor Carron's regimen involves starting the patient on 250 mg. valproate 3 times daily, increasing to 500 mg. 3 times daily along with an antidepressant if the antidepressant does not work by itself. Transsacral nerve blocks of usually the S3 nerve root with 0.25 per cent bupivacaine and subsequent 6 per cent aqueous phenol provided relief to 53 per cent of 15 patients for an average of 26.5 months.[7]

Finally, Doctor Carron noted that one should attempt multimodality treatments and then worry later about why they work. He indicated that narcotics worked better for somatic pain than for autonomic or visceral pain. They may affect the affective component more than the sensory aspect. He also noted that transsacral neurolysis may be combined with drug treatment. Biofeedback and acupuncture were not discussed.

Dr. David T. Schwartz discussed the psychological aspects of interstitial cystitis. He began with an apology to interstitial cystitis patients as having been unfairly stigmatized by the psychological and psychiatric profession. He noted that there was no database relating psychological variables to interstitial cystitis symptoms and that a diagnosis of exclusion without positive findings is not necessarily psychological. Most patients have difficulty in coping with the fact that no one seems to care whether they suffer without any explanation of the problem. This is one of the major problems with interstitial cystitis patients and it is one of the needs that the Interstitial Cystitis Association satisfies. How is hysteria diagnosed from a reaction to being told that "there is nothing that you can do"? It is difficult. There is no evidence for the relationship of specific personality traits in specific diseases but there is evidence to suggest a disease-prone personality. He suggested a biopsychosocial model of the development of interstitial cystitis. Life stress plus lack of coping resources plus genetic vulnerability plus something happening (infection or another event) is the initiation. This gives rise to immune suppression, which gives rise to interstitial cystitis pathogenesis, which gives rise to symptoms. The symptoms then cause hyperattentiveness to bladder distension, which gives rise to a pattern of increased frequency and a decrease in average bladder distension, and the patient then seeks help from the medical system. The lack of diagnosis and support gives rise to increased stress. These patients may well have a bladder that never allows itself to fill. Doctor Schwartz noted that other things could be done with psychology than treating the patient for a hysterical disorder. Psychological/behavioral interventions include patient compliance (reassurance, education, regular followup and group support), stress-mediated aspects (cognitive – behavioral treatment, training in relaxation and biofeedback) and bladder distension (education and biofeedback-aided behavioral training to increase capacity). He considers interstitial cystitis to be a physical disorder with psychological consequences that vary from patient to patient. Finally, he noted that it would help greatly if a physician was able to say "there is something wrong with you, but I cannot diagnose it or help it with conventional therapy".

In section 6 Dr. Merete Holm-Bentzen discussed the diagnosis of interstitial cystitis. She considers interstitial cystitis to be a part of the painful bladder syndrome. Painful bladder is divided into known and unknown etiologies. Diagnosis is made on the basis of history, symptoms, signs, cystoscopy, urodynamic studies, histology and laboratory tests. Radiology has a limited role, if any. Painful bladder breaks down mainly into classical interstitial cystitis (defined by 20 mast cells or more per mm.^{3}), eosinophilic cystitis and detrusor myopathy. Cystoscopy is performed at 80 cm. water pressure with distension at 1 minute with the patient under anesthesia. This was agreed upon later as a reasonable standardized way to perform cystoscopy and distension. Deep biopsies were taken by Doctor Holm-Bentzen. It should be noted that her patients with interstitial cystitis included those with detrusor instability, although she characterized these as having "slight" detrusor instability. Detrusor instability means involuntary bladder contraction without detectable neurological disease. Later, we had agreed to exclude these patients from those undergoing clinical studies. One of the interesting points made, and one of the reasons why her views on mast cells seem to have changed with time, was that of patients who underwent repeat biopsy only 26 had the same diagnosis, while 32 had 2 different diagnoses, 6 had 3 and a smaller number had 4. She admits that this casts doubt regarding the value of histopathology in the diagnosis of interstitial cystitis. Laboratory diagnosis should include a negative urine culture and negative cytology study. One can perform blood tests for autoimmunity. Eosinophilic cationic protein is released when mast cells are degranulated and is increased in patients with mastocytosis. This can be used as a marker. 1,4- Methyl imidazol acetic-acid is a metabolite of histamine that also is increased in mastocytosis and can be used as a marker. Epidermoid growth factor, which increases the production of glycosaminoglycans, shows no difference in interstitial cystitis patients versus control patients. As far as analysis of the glycosaminoglycans layer is concerned, it is convenient to postulate some abnormality, either qualitative or quantitative. Electron microscopy seems to show no difference in appearance but Doctor Holm-Bentzen concedes that there may be a permeability difference.

Doctor Fall and associates discussed the diagnosis of interstitial cystitis in Sweden.[8] Doctor Fall considers this an uncommon disease with no uniform classification whose diagnosis is made later. He also considers the primary symptom as pain radiating to the groin or related to bladder filling and he believes that this pain should be rated as severe, moderate or mild. The degree of frequency should be evaluated with a micturition chart greater than 48 hours in duration. These patients typically have fixed low volumes. Endoscopically, he finds a classical ulcer in most patients. These ulcers rupture with distension and cause petechial bleeding with further distension. After distension there is slight bullous edema. In the nonulcerative form, as he describes it, there is only glomerulation and petechial bleeding. Pathological findings include a mononuclear infiltrate and an increase in connective tissue mast cells. Muscularis and lamina propria mast cells increase greatly in the ulcerative type of interstitial cystitis. Mast cells in the muscularis are increased somewhat in the nonulcerative form but not in the lamina propria. Doctor Fall believes that the typical symptoms must include symptoms at least 2 years in duration, nocturia equal to or greater than 3, suprapubic discomfort or pain relieved partially or completely by voiding, a negative urine culture and no other symptoms of bladder disease.

It should be noted that there is at least considerable question about what Doctor Fall considers to be an ulcer. It was stated later that perhaps some sort of an atlas should be published representing a consensus as to what people believe represents an ulcer versus a scar that splits with distension to cause submucosal bleeding, versus simply coalesced areas of hemorrhage, versus true glomerulation.

Doctor Fall presented his experience with transcutaneous electrical nerve stimulation and transurethral resection in the treatment of interstitial cystitis. Electrical stimulation was applied suprapubically with low and high frequencies (trial and error) and intermittently for 2 hours twice daily. A gradual positive result was noted, when one occurred, with the first effect being noted only after 2 to 6 weeks, a good effect being noted after 2 to 3 months and the fact that a maximum effect may take up to a year. In terms of ulcerative and nonulcerative disease he noted an excellent result in 4 patients within 1 month, a good result in 12 within 1 month and a poor result in 4 within 13 months. It is difficult to explain why in the nonulcerative group the results were worse than one would expect with a placebo. In regard to transurethral resection for interstitial cystitis, Doctor Fall has treated 49 patients with an initial decrease in pain. He noted that pain is controlled better than frequency. The results were divided interestingly. A lasting effect was noted in 18 patients after 1 transurethral resection, 11 after 2 resections and 3 after 3 or 4 resections. In 12 patients there was no lasting effect after more than 2 resections. Five patients had 1 resection and the followup was too short. These patients had resectable areas of what he called ulcers but that looked like simply coalesced areas of hemorrhage on the slide.

Dr. C. Lowell Parsons discussed his studies on sodium pentosanpolysulfate and noted that 60 per cent of the patients became "better". He indicated that symptomatic improvement sometimes is different from statistical improvement and that it is difficult to gauge improvement in patients with the urgency/frequency syndrome. In those who were treated successfully the average functional increase in bladder capacity was only 32 cc per void.

Doctor Parsons feels strongly that in interstitial cystitis the epithelial surface is not fulfilling its purpose. Glycosaminoglycans inhibit the adherence of bacteria, microcrystals, protein and tumour cells. Biochemical inactivation of the antiadherence property of the epithelial surface occurs in response to protamine, cyclomate, aspartane, saccharin and hydroxyanthralic acid. In his studies Doctor Parsons used pentosanpolysulfate at a dose of 100 mg. 3 times daily. In 1 study with oral drugs there was a 47 per cent drug response versus a 22 per cent good placebo response. He then switched to injection therapy, with 100 mg. injected subcutaneously 3 times a week. The responses were 30 per cent in the drug group and 7 per cent in the placebo group.

Interstitial cystitis patient accrual form

Automatic exclusions:
  <18 yrs. old
  Benign or malignant bladder tumors
  Radiation cystitis
  Tuberculous cystitis
  Bacterial cystitis
  Vaginitis
  Cyclophosphamide cystitis
  Symptomatic urethral diverticulum
  Uterine, cervical, vaginal or urethral Ca
  Active herpes
  Bladder or lower ureteral calculi
  Waking frequency <5 times in 12 hrs.
  Nocturia <2 times
  Symptoms relieved by antibiotics, urinary antiseptics, urinary analgesics (for example
     phenazopyridine hydrochloride)
  Duration <12 mos.
  Involuntary bladder contractions (urodynamics)
  Capacity >400 cc, absence of sensory urgency
Automatic inclusions:
  Hunner's ulcer
Pos. factors:
  Pain on bladder filling relieved by emptying
  Pain (suprapubic, pelvic, urethral, vaginal or perineal)
  Glomerulations on endoscopy
  Decreased compliance on cystometrogram

Bladder distension is defined arbitrarily as 80 cm. water pressure for 1 minute. Two positive factors are necessary for inclusion in the study population. Substratification at the conclusion of the study by bladder capacity with the patient under anesthesia was less than and greater than 350 cc.

Doctor Holm-Bentzen presented the results of her treatment with subcutaneous heparin for interstitial cystitis. Heparin stabilizes mast cells, antagonizes histamine, bradykinin and prostaglandin E and inhibits the complement system and action of inflammatory agents. Doctor Holm-Bentzen cited the preliminary study by Lose in which patients were treated with 5,000 units subcutaneously 3 times a day for 2 days and then twice a day for 5 to 7 days. This study only included 7 female and 1 male patients who had had symptoms for 6 years, 4 of whom had increased mast cells. In 5 of 8 patients the pain was gone, in 2 it was reduced and 1 showed no change. Nocturia did not disappear in any patient but it was reduced in 5 and showed no change in 3. Daytime frequency was reduced in 7 patients and showed no change in 1. Eosinophilic cationic protein decreased by day 2. Doctor Holm-Bentzen performed a double-blind study in female patients with interstitial cystitis symptoms more than 1 year in duration. All patients had petechial bleeding on cytoscopy and all had increased eosinophilic cationic protein. There were 15 patients with greater than 28 and 15 with less than 28 mast cells per mm.[3]. They were treated with 5,000 units 3 times daily for 2 days, twice daily for 5 days and then once daily for 7 days. One patient dropped out, 20 patients were treated with heparin and 18 received placebo. There was no difference in the placebo and heparin treated groups. Pain decreased in both groups.

The consensus criteria for diagnosis of interstitial cystitis are presented in the table. The purpose of these criteria is not to define the disease but to ensure that in any group studies that adhere to these inclusion and exclusion criteria the populations will be relatively comparable. It is assumed that virtually all of these patients will present with symptoms of urgency and what they consider frequency, and so these are not included as positive factors or as an absolute inclusion factor.

Jay Y. Gillenwater
Department of Urology
University of Virginia School of Medicine
Charlottesville, Virginia
    and
Alan J. Wein
Division of Urology
Hospital of the University of Pennsylvania
Philadelphia, Pennsylvania

References

1. Bourque, J. P.: Surgical management of the painful bladder. J. Urol., **65:** 25, 1951.
2. Hunner, G. L.: A rare type of bladder ulcer in women: report of cases. Boston Med. Surg. J., **172:** 660, 1915.
3. Messing, E. M. and Stamey, T. A.: Interstitial cystitis: early diagnosis, pathology and treatment. Urology, **12:** 381, 1978.
4. Walsh, A.: Interstitial cystitis. In: Campbell's Urology, 4th ed. Edited by J. H. Harrison, R. F. Gittes, A. D. Perlmutter, T. A. Stamey and P. C. Walsh. Philadelphia: W. B. Saunders Co., vol. 1, chapt. 19, pp. 693–707, 1978.
5. Oravisto, K. J.: Epidemiology of interstitial cystitis. Ann. Chir. Gynaec. Fenn., **64:** 75, 1975.

6. Aldenborg, F., Fall, M. and Enerbäck, L.: Proliferation and transepithelial migration of mucosal mast cells in interstitial cystitis. Immunology, **58**: 411, 1986.
7. Simon, D. L. Carron, H. and Rowlingson, J. C.: Treatment of bladder pain with transsacral nerve block. Anesth. Analg., **61**: 46, 1982.
8. Fall, M., Johansson, S. L. and Aldenborg, F.: Chronic interstitial cystitis: a heterogeneous syndrome. J. Urol., **137**: 35, 1987.

A small workshop on interstitial cystitis was held under the auspices of NIDDK on 22 November 1988, primarily to present 1-year test results of the preliminary diagnostic criteria which had been established for IC at the 1987 workshop. It should be emphasized that these criteria were originally designed *not* to "diagnose" IC, but to select out a population of IC patients that would be about 90% consistent from the series of one physician to another. The criteria were designed to select a population for study of IC, the feeling being reasonably certain that all patients selected by these criteria would indeed have what most would agree upon was "the disease", recognizing that some patients who have been diagnosed might not in fact be selected under these criteria. Following presentations by Lowell Parsons (University of California at San Diego), Philip Hanno (University of Pennsylvania), and Grannum Sant (Tufts University), it was decided that the criteria needed to be modified, lest 20%–40% of patients in various series who had been diagnosed as having IC be excluded. The following criteria were those decided by the workshop participants as those which would be applied to patients to be enrolled in *research studies* on IC.

To be included as IC, patients must have either glomerulations on cystoscopic examination or a classic Hunner's ulcer, and they must have either pain associated with the bladder or urinary urgency. Examination for glomerulations should occur after distension of the bladder under anesthesia to 80–100 cm of water pressure for 1–2 min. The bladder may be distended up to two times before evaluation. The glomerulations must be diffuse – present in at least three quadrants of the bladder – and there must be at least ten glomerulations per quadrant. The glomerulations must not be along the path of the cystocope (to eliminate artifact from contact instrumentation). The presence of any one of the following criteria will exclude the diagnosis of interstitial cystitis:

1. Bladder capacity of greater than 350 ml on awake cystometry using either gas or liquid as a filling medium
2. Absence of an intense urge to void with the bladder filled to 100 ml of gas or 150 ml of water during cystometry, using a fill rate of 30–100 ml/min
3. The demonstration of phasic involuntary bladder contractions on cystometry using the fill rate described above
4. Duration of symptoms less than 9 months
5. Absence of nocturia
6. Symptoms relieved by antimicrobials, urinary antiseptics, anticholinergics, or antispasmodics (musculotropic relaxants)
7. A frequency of urination, while awake, of less than eight times per day
8. A diagnosis of bacterial cystitis or prostatitis within a 3-month period
9. Bladder or lower ureteral calculi
10. Active genital herpes
11. Uterine, cervical, vaginal, or urethral cancer

12. Urethral diverticulum
13. Cyclophosphamide or any type of chemical cystitis
14. Tuberculous cystitis
15. Radiation cystitis
16. Benign or malignant bladder tumors
17. Vaginitis
18. Age less than 18 years

It is obvious that what has been left out (on purpose) of these criteria is any mention of specific pathologic findings on biopsy. There is no requirement for even a general type of inflammatory response, nor for any specific type of inflammatory or other marker cells, such as mast cells. Although patients satisfying these criteria would not be accepted into various European series as IC patients, it was felt that, at this time, there did not exist even a general consensus as to a minimal number of pathologic criteria which would permit a specific diagnosis of IC. This is obviously an area that needs further research. Is there a defined natural history of IC and are there developmental stages? Is there really an early and late form of the disease, and does one progress to the other? What is the role of the mast cell, if any, in pathophysiology and in diagnosis? Is detrusor mastocytosis a phenomenon specific for IC or does it exist in other forms of inflammation or bladder pathology? Although in the past it is clear that we were too restrictive in our diagnosis of IC, we must take great care that, in our efforts to help this significantly affected group of patients, we do not overdiagnose IC and make the term as meaningless as the current usage of "the urethral syndrome". Perhaps a formulation like that of Holm-Bentzen (and others), in which IC is considered a more specific category of a more general and amorphous diagnosis, such as painful bladder syndrome, makes more logical sense, although the criteria upon which that more specific diagnosis is made obviously have yet to be agreed upon. Certainly when reading a typical European or Scandinavian article about IC, it is quite easy to ascertain exactly which patient population the article concerns. Unfortunately, in the American literature, it is all too common to read an article about the diagnosis or treatment of IC, when in fact what one is reading about are the characteristics of and results from a group of patients that that author has diagnosed, in his or her practice, as having IC on the basis of a very general symptom complex that he or she has gotten used to.

Finally, what are the other potential areas that need to be investigated, from the standpoint of pathophysiology, diagnosis, and treatment, for the group of patients that are diagnosed as having IC?

1. As IC is primarily a sensory syndrome, we must fill the very large gaps in our knowledge of bladder sensory physiology. We know little about sensory receptors in the bladder, and especially those that subverse urgency and pain, about sensory neurotransmitters, and about the characteristics of the sensory afferents from the lower urinary tract. With such knowledge, it may be possible to develop pharmacologic antagonists which function at various levels in the afferent transmission of noxious impulses from the lower urinary tract. Capsaicin cream is already being tested as a treatment for the symptoms of herpetic neuralgia. One can certainly envision the application of similar concepts to the lower urinary tract. The concept of so-called neurogenic inflammation and

the involvement of primary afferent neurons in releasing neuropeptides which initiate inflammatory changes is an interesting one, and may have direct relevance to syndromes such as IC. These neuropeptides include not only substance P, but vasoactive intestinal polypeptide, neurokinin A, and calcitonin G-related peptide.

2. Is there a role of the arachiodonic acid pathway, the substrate for the synthesis of the mediators of inflammatory processes (prostaglandins and leukotrienes), in the development of the inflammatory response associated with IC? Is there a lack of an inhibitory substance or substances or is there an excess of a stimulus or promoter?

3. Whatever the final common pathway in the inflammatory response and in the generation of the afferent nociceptive impulses, do factors in the urine of these patients contribute to the pathophysiology? Can these or other factors in the urine of IC patients be used in diagnosis or in subcategorization?

4. One working hypothesis for pathophysiology involves the disruption of a normally protective glycosaminoglycan (GAG) layer on the transitional epithelium of the bladder. In theory this would permit toxic substances to initiate and perpetuate an inflammatory response in the deeper layers of the bladder. Current quantitative methods have detected no such abnormality; however, a qualitative defect is certainly possible, and, if this theory has merit, certainly these concepts can be used as a starting point for the development of preventive and therapeutic measures.

5. Although current studies have been unable to confirm IC as an immunologically mediated phenomenon, in the absence of a known cause, we should not overlook this as a possibility, and should concentrate efforts on more exact immunologic phenotyping of the bladder response. Similarly, although infection does not seem to be involved in pathogenesis, it may be that this area, too, has not been as completely investigated as it should be.

6. Is there value to exhaustively studying the bladders of individuals who have experienced a clinical remission, either spontaneous or secondary to treatment? The obvious risk would be a re-exacerbation of symptomatology, but it may be that important differences might be found that would lead to a better understanding of pathophysiology. These studies do not necessarily mean biopsy only, but could include the utilization of various non-invasive modalities capable of looking at changes which are other than structural ones, such as magnetic resonance imaging and positron emission tomographic scanning.

Chapter 2

Historical Perspectives

A. Walsh

Interstitial cystitis was well recognized as a pathologic entity in the last century. For the nineteenth-century pathologist an interstitial inflammation was one in which edema and the cells of chronic inflammation were found in the interstitial tissue and thus distinguished from parenchymal disease. The best example of that distinction today persists in the kidney, where we still talk of glomerulonephritis and interstitial nephritis. The concept of interstitial inflammation also implied that the entire interstitial tissue was involved. Skene, in 1887, wrote "when the disease has destroyed the mucous membrane partly or wholly and extended to the muscular parietes, we have what is known as interstitial cystitis . . ." It is important to keep clearly in mind that the term "interstitial cystitis" does no more and no less than define a pathologic condition that may very well be the common end result of many different disease processes just as interstitial nephritis may be the result of conditions as diverse as bacterial pyelonephritis and drug nephropathy. It is clear that an interstitial cystitis can be caused by tuberculosis, schistosomiasis, cyclophosphamide and radiation. What we are concerned with in this volume is nonspecific interstitial cystitis – at least it is nonspecific in the present state of our knowledge.

Any discussion of the history of our knowledge of the disease must give a very important place to Hunner. Although he was by no means the first to describe the condition, Hunner must receive all the credit for drawing attention to interstitial cystitis. We must realize that in the first part of this century the very best cystoscopes available gave a very poorly defined and ill-lit view of the fundus of the bladder. It is not very surprising that when Hunner saw red and bleeding areas high on the bladder wall he thought that these areas were ulcers. The pseudonym "Hunner's ulcer" has been doubly unfortunate. It led people to think that the disease might be focal and not, as in fact it is, a pancystitis, and it also led physicians to look for an ulcer at cystoscopy and when no ulcer was found the diagnosis was missed. The term "Hunner's ulcer" must be abandoned because it is so seriously misleading. However, we should remember that Hunner applied the important epithet "elusive" to the disease (Hunner 1918). This epithet is totally justified. At cystoscopy the bladder may look virtually normal during the first filling and it is only when the bladder is viewed from empty to full a second time that the characteristic endoscopic appearances are manifest. It is a tribute to Hunner that in the 70 or so years since his description of the histology very little of consequence has been added until the recent emphasis on the importance of the mast cell (see Chap. 9).

The etiology remains a mystery. The earlier literature is full of accounts of attempts to incriminate microbiologic agents whether bacteria, viruses or fungi – so far with no success. Powell, in 1945, argued cogently that lymphatic obstruction was important, but there is no real evidence that this is so.

In recent times attention has focussed on the idea that interstitial cystitis might be an autoimmune disease. Indeed, Jokinen et al., in 1972, concluded that interstitial cystitis belonged to that group of autoimmune diseases in which the disease is restricted to one organ, whereas the autoantibodies are nonorgan specific. There is still a great deal of debate on this subject and it is far from proven that the disease is, in fact, autoimmune.

The relationship of the disease to neurosis has been discussed extensively. In 1944, Pool and Rives remarked that the patients were often considered neurotic, looked neurotic and that they wandered from doctor to doctor. It is extremely difficult in such patients as seem neurotic to know whether the disease caused the neurosis or the neurosis caused the disease in some way as acute stress can initiate and exacerbate ulcerative colitis. It is characteristic of patients with interstitial cystitis that they do go from doctor to doctor, ever more desperately seeking relief of the distressing symptoms. Very many such patients have been given both diagnoses and treatments varying from the inappropriate to the bizarre. While there is some evidence that the disease occurs more frequently in those with a nervous instability, we would do well to remember always what T. Leon Howard wrote in 1944: "I have not placed any significance on the nervous, whiney character of those females for I feel sure that if I had suffered as they had I would be both nervous and whiney also, except probably to a *greater degree*".

After the pioneer publications by Hunner the next really important study was the report in 1949 by Hand of 223 cases, including 204 women and 19 men. This very curious, approximately 11:1, female to male sex incidence is identical to that found by Oravisto in 1975 in a magnificent epidemiologic study conducted in an area of Finland with a population of about 1 million. This study remains unique but its conclusions are worth looking at in some detail as they correspond very closely with the experience in many other parts of the world. Oravisto found 18 cases of the disease in every 100 000 women in this special population. The ratio of women to men was a little over 10:1 and severe cases accounted for only 1 in 10 of all the patients. There was some evidence that the incidence had been increasing during the past decade. A most interesting feature of the Finnish study was the discovery that the disease does not as a rule progress continuously but reaches its final stage for a given patient rapidly, then remains at a constant level. The excellent studies of the Finnish group of Alfthan, Jokinen and Oravisto are among the most important contributions of recent times to our factual knowledge of interstitial cystitis (Oravisto et al. 1970).

One striking feature of the histology that has received little attention from the researchers is the abundance of nerve tissue in some areas, as first described by Hand in 1949. In some cases the nerves lie just below the margin of the subepithelial reaction and in others they penetrate it. While the nerves in the deeper structures are intact, those in the areas of subepithelial reaction have lost their sheaths, giving the impression of a proliferation of nerve tissue. It is interesting to speculate that these nerves may, in fact, be vipergic.

When we come to look at the history of treatment we find what I have elsewhere termed an extraordinary gallimaufry of pills, potions and procedures. The great variety of remedies probably reflects not only guesses about etiology but also despairing efforts to relieve the distress of patients suffering from a condition that was very poorly understood. Systemic drugs are largely ineffective. There has been some measure of success with anti-inflammatory agents such as orgotein (Marberger et al. 1974) and benzydamine (Walsh 1976), chloroquine and azathioprine (Oravisto and Alfthan 1976), but the results were too patchy. A curious feature of these few occasionally effective drugs was that they gave an all or none response. There was either very good relief or no effect at all. In view of the fact that there are still patients who are given steroids it is worth emphasizing that despite many enthusiastic early reports there is not a single report of good long-term results with steroid therapy. There would seem to be no justification whatever for subjecting a patient with interstitial cystitis to the very considerable risks associated with prolonged treatment with steroids.

The first significant step in treatment was made by Bumpus when, in 1930, he advocated distension of the bladder under anesthesia. This always gives considerable temporary relief from pain. Endoscopic maneuvers such as infiltration of the bladder wall with various drugs and transurethral resection and fulguration may, in fact, owe their effect to the bladder distension that is involved in such a procedure. Any future studies of the efficacy of these transurethral techniques should be controlled by comparison with patients whose bladders are distended in the same way and for the same period of time as the group operated on. As yet, we have no information as to whether or not the degree and duration of bladder distension makes a significant difference, but I have personal experience of two patients who had a vastly better response to Helmstein balloon distension for 6 hours than they previously had to simple bladder distension.

Many different instillations into the bladder have been tried. There are very conflicting reports about the value of oxychlorosene (Clorpactin). There are many favourable reports about the use of intravesical dimethyl sulfoxide (DMSO) as advocated by Stewart et al. in 1967.

Because pain is such a severe and dominant symptom it is natural that surgical denervation should have been tried. According to Learmonth (1931), this was first suggested by Jaboulay in 1899. It is quite clear that presacral neurectomy is of no value. Bilateral division of the third sacral nerve as advocated in 1956 by Moulder and Meirowsky seemed very successful in the few cases in which it was tried, and there would certainly seem to be eminent justification for further trial of selective sacral neurectomy.

Turner-Warwick postulated that the success of enterocystoplasty might, in fact, be due to bladder denervation, and he devised two operations, cystocystoplasty and cystolysis, to achieve supratrigonal denervation (Turner-Warwick and Handley-Ashken 1967; Worth and Turner-Warwick 1973). However, the long-term results of these procedures are poor and there is a very significant risk of bladder contraction.

Bladder substitution surgery in the form of enterocystoplasty does have a great deal to offer. Many authors have written enthusiastically about the excellent results of enterocystoplasty in the treatment of interstitial cystitis. One reason that the operation is not more widely used is the general misconception about the true purpose of the procedure. In the treatment of interstitial cystitis, the object of enterocystoplasty is not *enlargement* but *replacement* of the diseased body of the bladder. Far too much stress has been laid on bladder capacity in this disease. Pain may be quite intolerable even though the bladder can be filled to 300, 400 or even 500 ml under anesthesia. The extreme frequency of micturition is, in most cases, a function of the severe pain of bladder filling. Genuine bladder contraction down to a very small capacity is in fact uncommon in interstitial cystitis. Any form of augmentation cystoplasty is doomed to failure. The entire bladder, except the trigone, must be removed. Any segment of bowel will do for replacement but by a long way the easiest to use is the cecum and ascending colon. We are now aware that such bowel segments should be detubularized.

Envoi

We have advanced little since Hanash and Pool wrote (in 1969): "The cause is unknown, the diagnosis is difficult, and treatment is temporary and palliative." What we now need above all are properly controlled studies in histologically proven cases – studies that so far are singularly lacking. This lack is not due to medical ineptitude but rather to the fact that any one center meets relatively few cases. There would seem to be a great need for some central organization to initiate and supervise multicenter studies.

References

Bumpus HC (1930) Interstitial Cystitis; its treatment by overdistension of the bladder. Med Clin North Am 13:1495

Hand JR (1949) Interstitial cystitis: report of 223 cases (204 women and 19 men.) J Urol 61:291–310

Hanash KA, Pool TL (1969) Interstitial cystitis in men. J Urol 102:427–428

Howard TL (1944) My personal opinions on interstitial cystitis (Hunner's ulcer). J Urol 51:526

Hunner GL (1918) Elusive ulcer of the bladder: further notes on a rare type of bladder ulcer with a report on 25 cases. Am J Obstet 78:374

Jokinen EJ, Alfthan OS, Oravisto KJ (1972) Antitissue antibodies in interstitial cystitis. Clin Exp Immunol 11:333

Learmouth JR (1931) Neurosurgery in the treatment of diseases of the urinary bladder. 2. Treatment of vesical pain. J Urol 26:13

Marberger H, Huber W, Bartsch G et al. (1973) Orgotein: A new anti-inflammatory metalloprotein drug. Evaluation of clinical efficacy and safety in inflammatory conditions of the urinary tract. Int Urol Nephrol (Budap) 6:61

Moulder MK, Meirowsky N (1956) The management of Hunner's ulcer by differential sacral neurotomy: preliminary report. J Urol 75:261

Oravisto KJ (1975) Epidemiology of interstitial cystitis. Ann Chir Gynaecol Fenn 64:75–77

Oravisto KJ, Alfthan OS (1976) Treatment of interstitial cystitis with immunosuppression and chlorquien derivatives. Eur Urol 2:82

Oravisto KJ, Alfthan OS, Jokinen EJ (1970) Interstitial cystitis: clinical and immunological findings. Scan J Urol Nephrol 4:37–42

Pool TL, Rives HF (1944) Interstitial cystitis: treatment with silver nitrate. J Urol 51:520

Powell TO (1945) Studies on the etiology of Hunner's ulcer. J Urol 53:823

Skene AJC (1887) Diseases of the bladder and urethra in women. William Wood, New York

Stewart BH, Persky L, Kiser WD (1967) The use of dimethyl sulfoxide (DMSO) in the treatment of interstitial cystitis. J. Urol 98:671

Turner-Warwick R, Handley-Ashken M (1967) The functional results of partial, sub-total and total cystoplasty with special reference to ureterocystoplasty, selective sphincterotomy and cystocystoplasty. Br J Urol 39:3

Walsh A (1976) Benzydamine – a new weapon in the treatment of interstitial cystitis. Trans Am Assoc Genitourin Surg 68:43

Walsh A (1978) Interstitial cystitis. In: Campbell's Urology, 4th edn., vol I. Saunders, Philadelphia, pp 693–707

Worth PHL, Turner-Warwick R (1973) The treatment of interstitial cystitis by cystolysis with observations on cystoplasty. Br J Urol 45:65

Section 2

Epidemiology and Etiology

Chapter 3

Epidemiology of Interstitial Cystitis: 1

K.J. Oravisto

Since my paper in 1975 (Oravisto 1975), very little has been published on the epidemiology of interstitial cystitis. The smallness of the various series and the difficulty of collecting pertinent data do not encourage general epidemiologic conclusions. Different statistics can be compared and combined only with great caution because of the variability of the diagnosis. Moreover, my own study cannot be easily repeated, because in the region where I collected my series the care of these patients nowadays is too dispersed.

Prevalence

The only existing statistics concerning a whole regional population is the above-mentioned study (Oravisto 1975). The diagnosis is based on the following findings:

1. Frequency and pain or feeling of discomfort uninterruptedly for months or years, despite sterile urine
2. Biopsy of a seemingly unaffected site of the bladder wall shows variable fibrosis, edema and/or lymphocytic infiltration
3. Overdistension is often followed by temporary relief of symptoms

In the province of Uusimaa in southern Finland, including the city of Helsinki, there were 974 305 inhabitants, with 523 794 women and 450 511 men. Women aged more than 20 years numbered 510 941. The inhabitants of rural communities numbered 251 570 and those of cities 721 925, including 523 051 inhabitants of Helsinki.

The number of patients living in this area at the time of diagnosis totalled 103, of whom 95 were women and 8 were men. There were no children as we do not treat children at our clinic. The prevalence of interstitial cystitis is given in Table 3.1. The number of men is too small for separate analysis.

Table 3.1. Prevalence of interstitial cystitis

Both sexes, all ages	10.6:100 000
Women, all ages	18.1:100 000
Women, in age group >20 years	18.6:100 000
Men: not calculated	

Incidence

In the 10-year period of 1962–71 64 patients were stricken with interstitial cystitis, of whom 61 were female (Oravisto 1975). Each year the disease was manifested in 4–8 patients. In the preceding decade 1952–61 the annual incidence was only 1–4 patients. It remains unclear whether there was a true increase of the incidence from the first decade to the second. After 1971, at least, no more increase seems to have occurred, although accurate figures cannot be presented. The annual incidence calculated from the years 1962–71 is presented in Table 3.2.

Table 3.2. Incidence of interstitial cystitis

Both sexes, all ages	0.66:100 000
Women, all ages	1.2:100 000
Women, in age group >20 years	1.3:100 000
Men: not calculated	

Sex

All authors agree that the great majority of interstitial cystitis patients are women. The percentage of men varies from 2% to 23%, the most frequent figure being about 10% (Kretschmer 1939; Higgins 1941; Hand 1949; Smith 1952; Burford and Burford 1958; Kinder and Smith 1958; von Garrelts 1966; Hanash and Pool 1969; Greenberg et al. 1974; Oravisto 1975; Stewart and Shirley 1976; de Juana and Everett 1977; Messing and Stamey 1978; Shirley and Mirelman 1978). In my own series there are 8% of male patients. The percentage of men in the combined series of all above-mentioned authors is 9.1%. The diagnostic acuity and selection of patients influence the sex ratio greatly. The great preponderance of women is typical of autoimmune diseases.

Age

The age distribution has apparently moved to older age because the correct diagnosis is often made several years after the actual onset of the disease. In

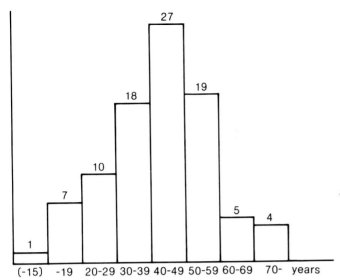

Fig. 3.1. Age distribution of 95 women at onset of interstitial cystitis, reported by Oravisto (1975).

Hand's material in 1949 the time lag was averaged 7–12 years. In our earliest series (Oravisto et al. 1970) the time lag was averaged 6 years, but now the median of the lag is 3–5 years depending on the severity of the disease. Most statistics are probably based on the age at the beginning of the treatment, which is preceded by an unstated length of time from the onset of illness.

The time of onset can in most cases be accurately inferred from the history of the patient. The time of onset is given in Hand's series (1949) and in my own (Oravisto 1975). Interstitial cystitis can begin at any age. The youngest patient in Hand's series was 13 years, and in my series the youngest patient was 11 years at the onset of continuous symptoms. Some large series of children (McDonald et al. 1958; Chenoweth and Clawater 1960; Geist and Antolak 1970) are not accepted by others (Farkas et al. 1977; de Juana and Everett 1977) as interstitial cystitis. The age distribution of my own material is shown in Fig. 3.1.

Menopause does not play a role in the etiology of the disease: in Hand's series the average age was 35.5 years in mild cases and 41 in severe cases and in my series more than one-third were younger than 40 years.

The age distribution of men seems to be largely similar to that of women. The data are not sufficient for a detailed study.

Severity Grades

The patients can be classified as mild and severe cases in spite of the diffuse and arbitrary definitions. Mild cases either do not progress to more severe at all or only after many years (Oravisto 1975; Messing and Stamey 1978). The percentage of mild cases is 31%–68% (Hand 1949; Oravisto 1975; Messing and Stamey 1978) and that of the very severe cases 10%–14%. Between these groups is the ill-defined group of moderately severe cases which cannot be distinguished from the mild group on clear objective grounds; however, the patients subjectively suffer decisively more and have more restrictions in their daily lives than the mild group.

Men belong to the mild group or sometimes to the moderately severe group but never to the very severe one.

Interstitial Cystitis in Urological Practice

In the light of the above facts the average urologist has constantly in his care several patients with mild or moderately severe interstitial cystitis. Truly severe cases are rare. In a region where urological expertise has been previously unobtainable he will rapidly accumulate a cohort of patients who have until now been treated as suffering from a chronic bacterial cystitis or psychiatric disorder (women) or a prostatic hyperplasia or so-called chronic prostatitis (men). Almost every year there will arise a fresh case of interstitial cystitis among his potential clients.

References

Burford EH, Burford CE (1958) Hunner ulcer of the bladder: a report of 187 cases. J Urol 79:952–955

Chenoweth CV, Clawater EW Jr (1960) Interstitial cystitis in children. J Urol 83:150–152

de Juana CP, Everett JC (1977) Interstitial cystitis. Experience and recent literature. Urology 10:325–329

Farkas A, Waisman J, Goodwin WE (1977) Interstitial cystitis in adolescent girls. J Urol 118:837–839

Geist RW, Antolak SJ Jr (1970) Interstitial cystitis in children. J Urol 104:922–925

Greenberg E, Barnes R, Stewart S, Furnish T (1974) Transurethral resection of Hunner's ulcer. J Urol 111:764–766

Hanash KA, Pool TL (1969) Interstitial cystitis in men. J Urol 102:427–428

Hand JR (1949) Interstitial cystitis: report of 223 cases (194 women and 19 men). J Urol 61:291–310

Higgins CC (1941) Hunner's ulcer of the bladder: (review of 100 cases). Ann Intern Med 15:708–715

Kinder CH, Smith RD (1958) Hunner's ulcer. Br J Urol 30:338–343

Kretschmer HL (1939) Elusive ulcer of the bladder: a report of 138 cases. J Urol 42:385–395

McDonald HP, Upchurch WE, Artime M (1958) Bladder dysfunction in children caused by interstitial cystitis. J Urol 80:354–356

Messing EM, Stamey TA (1978) Interstitial cystitis: early diagnosis, pathology, and treatment. Urology 12:381–392

Oravisto KJ (1975) Epidemiology of interstitial cystitis. Ann Chir Gynaecol Fenn 64:75–77

Oravisto KJ, Alfthan OS, Jokinen EJ (1970) Interstitial cystitis: clinical and immunological findings. Scand J Urol Nephrol 4:37–42

Shirley SW, Mirelman S (1978) Experiences with colocystoplasties, cecocystoplasties and ileocystoplasties in urologic surgery; 40 patients. J Urol 120:165–168

Smith GG (1952) Interstitial cystitis. J Urol 67:903–915

Stewart BH, Shirley SW (1976) Further experience with intravesical dimethyl sulfoxide in the treatment of interstitial cystitis. J Urol 116:36–38

von Garrelts B (1966) Interstitial cystitis: thirteen patients treated operatively with intestinal bladder substitutes. Acta Chir Scand 132:436–443

Chapter 4

Epidemiology of Interstitial Cystitis: 2

P.J. Held, P.M. Hanno, A.J. Wein, M.V. Pauly and
M. A. Cahn

Introduction

The urology literature has voluminous articles bearing on the epidemiology of
interstitial cystitis (IC). For example, the Hanno and Wein (1987) review of IC
cites 12 articles; Messing's (1984) chapter on IC in Campbell's textbook (1984)
cites 19. Yet the epidemiology literature is summarized in just a few paragraphs.
Messing (1984) used two paragraphs; Walsh's review in an earlier Campbell's
textbook (1978) also used only two; Hanno and Wein (1987) were more
expansive and used four paragraphs. One reason for the brevity is that with the
exception of Oravisto (1975) nearly all the literature made reference only in
passing to the issue of epidemiology.

This chapter will follow a different approach. It will review much of the past
literature but will also present, in some detail, new material from a study whose
total focus was the epidemiology of IC. This study was produced in the summer
of 1987 as part of the National Institutes of Health Workshop on Interstitial
Cystitis.[1] The new material was based on data from four sources:

1. A random survey of 127 board certified urologists who supplied material on
   prevalence and incidence of IC, and criteria they used in diagnosing IC. This
   sample is called *BCU*.[2]

---

[1] National Institute of Diabetes and Digestive and Kidney Diseases (NIDDK), Division of Kidney,
Urologic and Hematologic Diseases, Workshop on Interstitial Cystitis held in Bethesda, Maryland,
on 28–29 August 1987. The study was designed and implemented by Philip J. Held, PhD, Philip M.
Hanno, MD, Alan J. Wein, MD, Mark V. Pauly, PhD, and Marjorie A. Cahn, MA. The study
received advice and strong support from Vicki Ratner, MD and Gary Striker, MD. Suzy Fletcher,
PhD contributed to the design of questionnaires. The study would not have been possible without
the support of the Interstitial Cystitis Association, The Urban Institute, and NIDDK.

[2] Additional responses were received subsequent to the analyses presented here. The samples were
increased as follows: BCU, 44; PD, 10; PT, 19; ICA, 99; GPOP, 10. These added responses will be
included in the publications in preparation.

2. A survey of 64 IC patients selected by the random sample of urologists. These patients were the last treated (called PT for *patient treated*) or last diagnosed (called PD for *patient diagnosed*). The sample was evenly divided between *PT* and *PD*.[2]

3. A survey of 902 female patients who were members of the Interstitial Cystitis Association and who reported a diagnosis of IC. This sample is called *ICA*.[2]

4. A random sample of 119 persons (73 females) from the US population. This sample is called *GPOP* for general population.[2]

The material from this study is still in preparation for publication (Hanno et al. 1990; Held et al. 1990a, b, c).

Prevalence and Incidence of Interstitial Cystitis

Any review of the literature on the prevalence (total number of cases) and incidence (new cases presenting per unit of time) of IC would suggest that little is known with any degree of certainty. Historically, IC was considered a rare disease (Hunner 1915). Oravisto (1975) reported that IC in the severe form is rare. Pool (1967) reported that many physicians claim to have never seen a case.

However, there are a number of articles which reported statistics that challenge this general wisdom. For example, Hand (1949) estimated that 4.79% of the patients he had seen had IC. Such an estimate would hardly qualify IC as a rare disease if this were generalizable to other urologists. More recently, Oravisto (1975) concluded "the disease is not rare when mild and moderately severe cases are diagnosed."

The range of estimates is very large. Messing (1984) cites a range of incidence estimates (new patients presenting per year) from 0.07% to 0.14% of all urology hospital admissions (Bowers ånd Lattimer 1957) and 0.25%–0.5% of new urology outpatients (von Garrelts 1966). While Messing (1984) comments that these estimates are "probably low" they are an order of magnitude smaller than Freiha and colleagues' (1980) estimate of 1.7%–4.2% of new urology outpatients. In fact there is no consensus on these issues. Messing (1984) summarizes by noting that "it is difficult to estimate its [IC's] actual incidence from literature."

By and large these past efforts have been based on purposive, i.e., nonrandom, nonpopulation-based studies. Frequently, the estimates are based on the authors' own practice or a selected clinic or hospital (Hand 1949; Carson 1953; Bowers and Lattimer 1957; Kinder and Smith 1958; von Garrelts 1966). Often, the terms "incidence" and "prevalence" are used interchangeably. As a consequence of these limitations, it is unwise to generalize from what may be anecdotal studies by authors who may or may not have had a representative urology practice.

A 1985 population-based study by the US National Center for Health Statistics estimates that there were 2.7 million visits in the USA to office-based physicians (roughly 80% of all physicians are office based) for all forms of cystitis (G. Gardocki 1987, personal communication). Chronic cystitis accounted for 9% of the total of 232 000 visits. If these chronic cystitis visits were for IC and if the average IC patient made 10 visits per year (as shown below, this is consistent with the IC patient surveys), this would imply a prevalence of 23 200 IC patients being seen by office-based physicians. However, since 80% of the total visits, i.e., another 2.2 million cystitis visits, were unspecified, in that no detail was given, this approach is not very precise either for chronic cystitis or IC.

In addition to the visits for cystitis, this same source reports 5.7 million visits per year for a diagnosis of urinary tract infections which would more than likely include some chronic cystitis and IC. Consequently, these population-based statistics might offer some upper bounds for estimating IC, but until the participating physicians are more specific in reporting their diagnoses, this source is not likely to lead to very precise estimates of IC.

One epidemiology study of IC in the urology literature does stand out from the rest in that it claims to be a population-based study which more readily justifies generalization to a larger universe. Oravisto's (1975)[3] study of IC for a population of approximately 1 million from the area of Helsinki, Finland is regarded as the most authoritative source for prevalence estimates of IC. Oravisto's 1975 estimates, based on 95 women and 8 men, were 18.1 cases per 100 000 females of all ages and 10.1 cases per 100 000 eligible population for both sexes. Oravisto also concludes that the ratio of females to males is 10:1. Extrapolated to the US 1985 population, the Oravisto estimate of prevalence would imply 21 500 females with IC.

The 1987 epidemiology study by Held et al. (1989c) used three separate methods to estimate the prevalence of female IC in the US. These three methods, all based on BCU, generated prevalence estimates of 19 400; 29 800; and 90 700 *diagnosed* female cases, with the average of the three being 43 500 female *diagnosed* cases.[4] When compared with the Oravisto prevalence rate, applied to the US female population, it is clear that the average of these three more recent estimates for the USA is higher by a factor of approximately two.[5]

It is also of interest that the Held et al. study showed that the women diagnosed as having IC by the sampled urologists, represented only one-fifth of

---

[3] Even here the issue of generalization is not beyond question. For example, Oravisto does not give evidence of why his study is population based. In his article (p 75) he states "we believe that we have included almost all the patients with interstitial cystitis in the city of Helsinki and in the surrounding administrative district of Uusimaa."

[4] The first two estimates were based on: the urologists' estimates of the proportion of their total patient load that was diagnosed female IC and the proportion of their reported cystitis visits that were diagnosed IC female. Combined with independent estimates (G Gardocki 1987, personal communication) of the total urology patient load and the total cystitis and urinary tract infection cases in the US for 1985, the IC patient prevalence is estimated. The third estimate is based on the sampled urologists' estimate of the total number of diagnosed IC females in their practice. Combined with the number of urologists in the US, the prevalence of diagnosed IC was estimated. The third estimate was given less weight in determining the average, given the likelihood of double counting of patients.

[5] The first two estimates of 19 400 and 29 800 are much closer to the Oravisto estimates. The average is pulled up by the third estimate of 90 700, which is based on a mean, across urologists, of 10.7 IC cases. The median was 5, which, if used instead of the mean, would have brought the third estimate down to 42 400 and an average of the three estimates to 30 900. This would imply a factor of 1.4 between these estimates and Oravisto's.

the cases that presented symptoms that were suggestive of IC.[6] These other cases were women whom the urologist classified as having "painful bladder syndrome and sterile, non-bacterial urine" but whom the urologist did not report as having been diagnosed with IC. While suggestive of IC, absence of the documentation of examination under anesthesia leaves the issue unsettled but of immense interest.

Oravisto's IC incidence estimate (new cases per year) for Finland was 1.2 new female cases per 100 000. Applying this estimate to the US population would yield approximately 1428 new female cases per year. Given approximately 7300 urologists in the US (Roback et al. 1986), this would suggest that only 20% of urologists would see a new female case each year, if each urologist diagnosed only one case. The study by Held et al. reported that at least 78% of the responding urologists had made a diagnosis of IC in the last year. Even if one assumes that each of these urologists made only one diagnosis in the last year (a conservative assumption), clearly the incidence implied by the Held et al. study for the USA in 1987 is higher than the estimate reported by Oravisto (Finland in 1975) by a factor of four. Again this would be a minimum, since it assumes that each of the urologists would be making only one diagnosis per year and other physicians none.

Other work by Held et al. used data from the US Medicare population to obtain estimates of the frequency of bladder dilation for interstitial cystitis.[7] They estimated in 1986, 8700 such procedures were performed on the elderly (over 65 years of age). This implies a rate of 30 per 100 000 population (male and female). While it is unknown what proportion of these procedures represented true positive new diagnoses, if only 20% were new incident cases, the incidence rate implied would be nine times Oravisto's estimated incidence for all age groups. Since the elderly represent approximately one- fifth of all IC cases (22% and 19% respectively for PD and PT samples), these estimates by Held et al., if substantiated by additional research, have dramatic implications for incidence estimates of the IC population. Specifically, these results suggest that Oravisto's estimates are too low for the US.

How does one interpret these higher estimates by Held et al. in light of Oravisto's prior estimates? First, the Oravisto estimates were for Finland in 1975. Generalization of these results to the USA in 1987 may not be warranted. Second, the estimates from Held et al. may have been biased if the responding urologists were physicians who had high IC patient loads and were consequently more interested in IC and more willing to respond to a voluntary study focused on IC. This latter explanation is called nonresponse bias. Third, definition of IC may be changing, i.e., the two studies may not be measuring the same population.

The first of these comments (USA versus Finland) may be impossible to evaluate with existing data. The second comment, i.e., the possibility that the Held et al. sample of responding urologists was not representative of the population of urologists, is plausible given that the response rate was only 26%. This issue has been addressed by a study of the nonresponding urologists and shows no such bias.

---

[6] The estimated ratio for "patients seen last week" was 4.9, with a standard error of 0.8. For "patients seen last month," the ratio was 5.5.

[7] Cystourethroscopy with dilation of bladder for IC with either local or general anesthesia.

The third point, i.e., the definition of IC may be changing, has been noted by others (Meares 1987). The criteria used by the responding urologists are discussed below, but in general would suggest that the criteria used by the US urologists are generally consistent with the Messing and Stamey (1978) triad of conditions: painful bladder, absence of infection or other causes, and glomerulation under endoscopic examination of the bladder following distension under general anesthesia. These criteria reported by the urologists are also consistent with those criteria developed by a consensus panel at the NIH/NIDDK workshop on IC in August 1987. These criteria are reproduced in an appendix (see pp. 46–47).

In support of these higher estimates it can be noted that Oravisto (1975) felt that his estimates were "minima" and that the "incidence has possibly been rising" in more recent years. Messing (1984) suggests that the estimates he cites are "low" and Meares (1987) raises the question of rising incidence rates.

In conclusion, there is not a consensus of findings or opinion on what the prevalence and incidence of IC are in the US. Although the Oravisto estimates of 1975 have generally been the accepted word, recent evidence by Held et al. (1989c) brings into question whether the Oravisto estimates for Finland in 1975 are directly relevant to the USA.

Beyond the rate of diagnosed IC there is the issue raised by Held et al. regarding possible undiagnosed IC, i.e., the painful bladder with sterile urine cases, that could possibly increase the estimates by a factor of five. This issue is discussed in the concluding section of this chapter (see pp. 42–46).

Diagnosis

In general, one of the difficulties in diagnosis of IC has been the multitude of symptoms and the lack of a clear etiology and pathogenesis of the disease. Oravisto et al. (1970) provided a set of diagnostic conditions. Messing and Stamey (1978) generated the triad of conditions, which include characteristic irritative voiding symptoms, the absence of objective evidence of other diseases that could cause these symptoms, and a typical cystoscopic appearance.

The work by Held et al. (1987a) showed that for 127 responding board-certified urologists, the criteria and methods they report using in diagnosing IC are, on average, reasonably close to the consensus of medical opinion as to the proper indicators of IC. (See Appendix for consensus criteria developed at the NIH/NIDDK 1987 workshop on IC.) These criteria, shown in Table 4.1, are ranked by average score from most often used to least often or never used. A score of 1.0 means that the urologists reported always or usually using that criterion or method; a score of 3.0 would mean that all urologists responded that they never or seldom used that criterion. For example, pain (suprapubic, pelvic, urethral, vaginal, perineal) was the single most commonly used criterion. It was ranked first, and had an average score of 1.24. On the other hand, rectal examination was the least used of the 28 methods, with an average score of 2.70.

Hypothesis tests by Held et al. showed that there was no evidence that urologist age was related to the criteria used to diagnose IC. In other words, there did not appear to be a difference in diagnostic technique between more

Table 4.1. Criteria used by board-certified urologists in diagnosing IC, 1987[a]

Rank	Score[b]	Criteria or methods
1	1.24	Pain (suprapubic/pelvic/urethral/vaginal/perineal)
2	1.27	Endoscopic examination under local anesthesia
3	1.32	Case history
4	1.40	Pain on filling relieved by emptying
5	1.42	Glomerulation under distension
6	1.47	Bladder biopsy (histopathology)
7	1.49	Urgency
8	1.50	Urine cultures
9	1.52	Hypersensitivity, pain, urgency or extreme discomfort on filling at liquid volume of <400 ml and gas volume of <300 ml
10	1.54	Hunner's ulcer
11.5	1.62	Mucosal hyperemia
11.5	1.62	Cystoscopy under general anesthesia
13	1.64	Duration of symptoms = >3 months
14.5	1.70	Response to therapy
14.5	1.70	Bloody effluent at endoscopy
16	1.71	Symptoms unrelieved by antibiotics, urinary antiseptics and urinary analgesics
17	1.76	Nocturia >2
18	1.78	Vaginal examination
19	1.79	Waking frequency = >5 times in 12 h with normal fluid intake
20	1.89	Physical examination of lower abdomen
21.5	1.98	Dysuria
21.5	1.98	Decreased compliance on cystometrogram
23	2.19	Feeling of incomplete emptying
24	2.46	Dyspareunia
25	2.58	Incontinence
26	2.62	Vaginal and cervical cultures
27	2.65	Hesitancy
28	2.70	Rectal examination

[a] n=127.
[b] Based on a three-point scale: 1.0, always or usually; 2.0, sometimes used; 3.0, never or seldom.

recent medical school graduates and earlier graduates. Similarly, given the size of the urologist's practice, Held et al. (1987a) reported no relationship between urologist's age and the number of diagnosed IC patients or the number of nondiagnosed IC female patients with painful bladder syndrome and sterile urine. These tests were additional indicators that board-certified urologists of more recent training appeared to diagnose IC in the same fashion as older members of the profession. If, for example, older urologists had a higher proportion of females with painful bladder and sterile urine symptoms, but not diagnosed IC, this could be taken as evidence that there were educational differences among urologists by age. However, this was not the case.

Patients Reports on Diagnosis of IC

Time to diagnosis is an issue of continuing controversy. Held et al. (1987a) reported that time between onset of symptoms and IC diagnosis differed according to patient sample (Table 4.2). The number of months varied from an

Table 4.2. Patient experiences before diagnosis of IC (females)[a]

Experiences	Results by sample	
Duration of symptoms	ICA	51 months
before diagnosis	PT	35 months
	PD	24 months
Number of physicians seen	ICA	4.9 physicians
before diagnosis	PT	3.4 physicians
	PD	2.2 physicians
Patients diagnosed	ICA	95%
by a urologist		
Symptoms fully manifested	ICA	33%
within 1 month of onset		

[a] Estimates are arithmetic means, except for percentages.

average of 24 months for the PD sample to 51 months for the ICA sample, with the PT sample falling in between with an average of 35 months. While these sample averages were all lengthy by any patient criteria, they were remarkably less than the averages reported by Oravisto (1975) of 6–7 years.

An interesting hypothesis which flows from this analysis is whether the time between symptoms and diagnosis might be getting shorter. Held et al. tested this hypothesis with the statistical data shown in Table 4.3. Conducting separate tests for the ICA sample and the samples of patients selected by the BCU, the null hypothesis of no difference between patients diagnosed before 1983 and after 1983 could not be rejected. While it could be argued that the PD and the PT sample (64 patients) might have been too small for adequate statistical power, this was not the case for the ICA sample of 902 patients.

Several sources have reported that IC patients typically go from physician to physician before a diagnosis is made (Pool 1967; Lapides 1975; Walsh 1978; Hanno and Wein 1987). Held et al. (1987a) reported that the number of physicians seen by a patient varied by sample, with the PD sample again reporting the lowest average of the three (see Table 4.2). The PD sample response was only 2.2 physicians on average, the ICA sample reported 4.9, and the PT sample again was in between with 3.4 physicians.

Table 4.3. Duration of symptoms before IC diagnosed, by year

Date of diagnosis and sample	Duration of symptoms in months[a]	n	P value[b]
PT and PD sample			
1983–1987	29.9	45	0.87
Pre–1983	32.0	13	
ICA sample			
1983–1987	51.1	566	0.96
Pre–1983	51.4	243	

[a] Arithmetic mean between onset and diagnosis.
[b] For the null hypothesis of a type 1 error of no difference using a two-tailed test.

While 95% of the ICA sample reported that a urologist made the diagnosis of IC, nearly all patients reported seeing other specialists before a diagnosis was made. The most common other specialists seen were gynecologists (70.9%), general or family practitioners (68.7%), and internists (35.2%).

Oravisto (1975) reported that the symptoms of IC typically progress rapidly to a final state with little worsening after that. Held et al. confirmed these basic patterns. One-third (32.5%) of their sample responded that time from onset to full manifestation was less than 1 month.

Table 4.4. IC symptoms as reported by patients (female)[a]

Symptom	Percentage of patients reporting	
	At onset	Now
Frequency, day	91	80
(average no. of times)	(18)	(15)
Nocturia	90	85
(average no. of times)	(7)	(5)
Pain	87	78
Pain relieved by voiding	59	57
Urgency	93	84
Stress incontinence	27	26
Burning with voiding	59	42
Difficulty emptying bladder	59	51
Difficulty starting flow	54	47
Retention of urine	45	42
Painful intercourse	63	57
Fluctuation during menstrual cycle (% Yes)	30%–48%	
Period(s) of remission (% Yes)	30%–46%	
Duration of remission (months)	Average 8 Range 1–80	

[a] ICA; PT and PD samples were similar.

Shown in Table 4.4 are the symptoms reported by all of the Held et al. patient samples, ranked by their frequency. Symptoms at onset and current symptoms are both displayed. These data suggest that the symptoms "now" are, on average, slightly less than at onset, i.e., there does not appear to be worsening of the symptoms.

Both Pool (1967) and Hand (1949) reported that female IC patients experienced fluctuation of the symptoms over the course of their menstrual cycle. Held et al. report that 30%–48% of their respondents report such fluctuations.

Periods of spontaneous remission have been reported by Pool (1967), Oravisto (1975) and Messing (1987). Held et al. reported that of the more recently diagnosed IC patients (PD), 30% had periods of spontaneous remission. For more established patients, the percentage was higher with 46%–50% reporting such remissions. The duration of these remissions varied substantially, with a range from 1 to 80 months, the average duration being 8 months.

Patient Demographics

It is generally agreed that IC is more characteristic of females than males, but even here there is some disagreement about the ratio. Hand (1949), Oravisto (1975) and De Juana and Everett (1977) all reported a female to male ratio of approximately 10:1. But Messing (1984), based on the literature (Oravisto 1975; Walsh 1978; Messing and Stamey 1978) quotes a difference of 6–11 times more common in females than in males. The Held et al. study sampled only females for the ICA cases, although the PD (last diagnosed) sample was at least 10% male, which would support the general wisdom. However, since the PD sample asked for females, i.e., selecting male respondents may have involved misunderstanding of instructions by the BCU, the 10% male estimate could be seen as a minimum.

Oravisto (1975) reports that IC can start at any age, although the most frequent age group is 30–59 years. Lapides (1975) reports that IC occurs more frequently in younger women than is commonly believed. More recently, Meares (1987) suggests that IC most commonly occurs in younger women. The work by Held (Table 4.5) shows a median age at onset of 40 (half the sample is above 40 and half below) for members of the ICA and recently diagnosed (PD) samples. The median age for the sample of patients recently treated (PT) in urologists' offices is 50 years, i.e., the IC patients who were previously diagnosed and seen by urologists more clearly resemble the Oravisto age experience than do the more recently diagnosed patients.

The distributions of age at onset for these three samples are shown in Fig. 4.1. The peak at age 50 for the PT sample, i.e., those patients recently treated, closely follows the Oravisto experience. However both the ICA and the PD

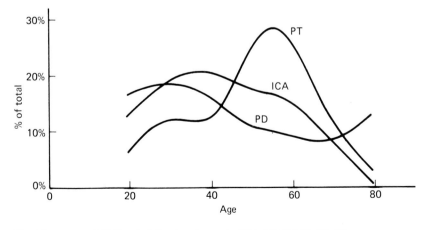

Fig. 4.1. at outset of IC (females).Numbers in sample: ICA, 886; PT, 32; PD, 28.

Table 4.5. Selected characteristics of IC patients (females)

Epidemiologic factors by sample	Estimate
Age at onset of IC symptoms	
Median (years)	
ICA, PD	40
PT	50
% less than 30 years old	
ICA, PD	26
PT	9
Mean years since onset	
ICA	6.0
PT	4.5
PD[a]	2.5
Education (years)	
All: ICA, PD, PT	13.5
GPOP (comparison)	13.8
Black (%)	
ICA	0.4
PT	0.0
PD	6.0
GPOP (comparison)	5.0
Jewish (%)	
ICA	14
PT	6
PD	3
GPOP (comparison)	3
Family income year, 1984–85 (median)	
ICA	$35 000
PT	34 000
PD	30 000
GPOP (comparison)	28 000
All US	28 000
Household size	
All: ICA, PD, PT	2.5
GPOP (comparison)	2.5
Currently married (%)	
All: ICA, PD, PT	77
GPOP (comparison)	75
All US[b]	61
Currently divorced (%)	
All: ICA, PD, PT	8
GPOP (comparison)	8
All US[b]	9
Number of different male sexual partners	
ICA	2.3
PT	1.4
PD	5.8
GPOP (comparison)	3.9
Childhood bladder problem	10–12 times more likely than GPOP group
All: ICA, PD, PT	($p < 0.01$), other covariates equal[c]
Urinary tract infections before inset	2 times more likely than GPOP group
of symptoms	($p < 0.01$), other covariates equal[c]
ICA, PD	

[a] Includes more recent observations.   [b] Females.   [c] Age, sex, education.

samples show a definite movement to a younger age consistent with the Meares (1987) comment. As shown in Table 4.5, both these samples had more than a fourth of their respondents aged less than 30 years at time of onset while only 9% of the PT sample was this young at time of onset. Oravisto (1975) reports an estimate in between, with one-fifth aged less than 30 years at time of onset.

Time since onset estimates (Table 4.5) show that ICA members have had IC the longest, with a mean of 6 years. The PT sample had a time of 4.5 years, and the PD sample, not surprisingly, had the shortest time of 2.5 years.

The educational level of the three samples of IC patients was quite similar at 13.5 years. This was similar to the estimate (13.8 years) for the national sample of respondents selected as a control group (GPOP).[8]

The prevalence of IC in blacks is uncertain, although the infrequency with which blacks with IC are encountered was commented on by Pool (1967), De Juana and Everett (1977) and Hanno and Wein (1987). One study from the Armed Forces Institute of Pathology reported by Smith and Dehner (1972) showed that 6 of 28 cases were black (21%), and half of these were male.

As reported in Table 4.5, both the ICA and the PT samples also had few blacks. The PD sample (recently diagnosed) showed however that 6% were black. This was almost identical to the 5% black from the control (GPOP) sample, although lower than the percentage of blacks in the US population as a whole.

To summarize the issue of race and IC prevalence it would appear that, like many other issues about IC, the prevalence of IC in black Americans is not clear. The actual cases seem rare enough for several authors to comment on it and yet there is enough evidence to preclude a ready assumption that IC does not occur in blacks. The data reported above suggest the issue should stay open and that further research is needed.

Also shown in Table 4.5 are some other statistics for IC patients from the work by Held et al (1987a). Family income for the ICA and the PT samples was definitely higher than the more recently diagnosed (PD) sample and the control sample (GPOP). The control sample was identical with the US population median at $28,000 per year. Household size was similar for all three samples of IC patients and the general population sample.

Pool (1967) remarks, in the context of dyspareunia, that divorce may be attributed to IC. The data in Table 4.5 show that the percentage married for all three samples of IC patients is quite similar to the GPOP comparison sample at 77% and 75%, respectively. This is apparently higher than that reported for US females (61%). The percentage divorced for all three samples is similar at 8%, which is somewhat lower than the US average for females. These statistics suggest that divorce is not likely to be attributed to IC.

Other statistics for IC patients are shown in Table 4.5. It has been suggested that IC may be linked to persons of Jewish origin (ICA 1987, personal communication). While the ICA and PT samples are somewhat more likely to be of Jewish origin (14% and 6%, respectively), the PD sample is similar to the comparison sample (GPOP), with approximately 3% Jewish. These data are inconclusive as to a link between IC and Jewish origin, although the data here

---

[8] This control sample is somewhat more highly educated than the US adult population which has less college (12.6 years of education) than the GPOP sample. (Statistical Abstract of the United States 1987).

show that the ICA sample is more likely to be Jewish than the population as a whole.

If IC were a sexually transmitted disease, one indicator might be that it would be correlated with the number of male sexual partners. As shown in Table 4.5, the number of male partners does not show an obvious pattern. Both the ICA and the PT samples (older with longer duration of disease) show fewer sexual partners than the comparison sample. Since the PD sample shows higher numbers than the comparison sample, it would appear that the issue should be left open for further analysis. A related issue for future analysis is whether there might be an age effect in these data since the PD sample may be younger than the control sample and sexual mores may have changed in the interim.

Hand (1949) records that 10% of his IC patients reported histories of childhood urinary problems. The work by Held et al. (1987a) reports substantially higher rates of childhood bladder problems. For the comparison sample, less than 2% responded positively to this question. For the three samples of IC patients, the percentages were: PD16%, PT 28%, ICA 21%. As shown in Table 4.5, even controlling for age, education, sample, and sex, the IC patients were 10–12 times more likely than the comparison sample to report childhood bladder problems.

It is of course possible that IC makes one more conscious of issues such as childhood bladder problems and therefore more likely to recall such issues in responding to a questionnaire. But it would seem that these data are at least consistent with the notion that children are not immune to IC (Geist and Antolak 1970; Lapides 1975; Farkas et al. 1977) and may be consistent with the reports of underdiagnosis for children (McDonald et al. 1958).

There are numerous reports linking IC to urinary tract infection (UTI) (Pool 1967; Messing 1984; Hanno and Wein 1987; Meares 1987). As shown in Table 4.5, both the ICA and the PD samples were twice as likely to report UTI than were the female respondents in the control sample. However, what is equally interesting is that a significant percentage of the IC patients (30%–42%) reported no UTI before the onset of IC. Further, for those IC patients who did report UTI before the onset of IC, a substantial portion of them had only one incident of UTI per year. In other words, over half of the IC patients report that they had fewer than one incident of UTI per year before the onset of IC.

Social and Economic Cost of IC

The cost of IC can be divided into two components: the direct cost of the medical care consumed in treatment and the various indirect costs. The latter includes losses due to the inability to work both in and out of the home, as well as other intangible but real costs such as pain and suffering. Held et al. showed that the medical cost of treating IC can be divided into the average cost per patient and the incremental cost of medical care consumed, as compared with what the patient would have consumed in the absence of IC. This latter is estimated by the consumption of medical care by a comparison sample of the US population (GPOP).

The average direct medical cost per IC per patient per year was estimated to be $3870. This estimate includes the cost of hospitals, physicians and drugs. With

Table 4.6. Economic cost of IC in the USA, 1987 [a]

Measure	Estimate
Cost per patient year:	
Average	$3870
IC-related incremental[a]	$2650
Total medical care cost per year @ 44 000 patients:	
Average ($/patient × 44k[b])	$170.3 mil
IC-related incremental[a]	$116.6 mil
IC-related lost economic production @ 44 000 patients:[b]	
Without wage "penalty"	$177.7 mil
With wage "penalty"	$311.7 mil

[a] k is 1000. Mil is million.
[b] Other covariates of age, sex, race, education held constant.

an estimated prevalence of 44 000 females the annual cost in the US would be $170.3 million.

This estimate inflates the cost of the disease since these patients would have had some medical care costs even in the absence of IC. Incremental costs in 1987 amount to $2650 per patient per year. These are the costs compared with a statistically matched sample of the US general population and include 125% more hospital days, and 206% more physician visits per year than an age, education and race matched sample of the general population. With a prevalence of 44 000 cases of IC, these incremental medical costs amount to $116.6 million per year.

Held et al. estimated that 24.9% of female IC patients were less likely to be working full time compared with a statistically matched (for age, sex, race and education) sample of the US population. This decrease in full-time work was partially offset by a 4.1% *increase* in the likelihood of working part time, again compared with a matched sample. It was also reported that IC patients who did work received $3.41 less per hour than did a matched sample of the general population. Using the national average wage rate for all females, the lost production would amount to $4039 per patient per year, without any wage reduction for those IC patients who did work. Including the IC wage rate "penalty" would increase the amount to $7084 per year. The total lost production, assuming a prevalence of 44 000, would amount to $177.7 million, or $311.7 million with the wage rate penalty. The average and incremental medical care costs per year, as well as indirect costs due to lost production, are shown in Table 4.6.

Direct medical cost and lost production are only part of the social cost of IC. Other measures of the cost impact of IC were reported by Held et al. (Table 4.7). IC patients were three to four times as likely to report thoughts of suicide as were a statistically matched sample of the general US population.[9] Women

[9] Held et al. estimated attempted suicide and found no statistical difference compared with the general population. However, their measure is likely to be biased low if, in fact, suicides are higher in the IC population. This is a classic case of non-response bias, i.e., if IC patients have a higher success rate than the general population, fewer such patients will be available to respond to the survey.

Table 4.7. Other social costs of IC[a]

| Measure | Relative to comparison group[a] | |
	Value[b]	P value[c]
Suicidal thoughts	ICA 3.85	(<0.01)
	PT 2.76	(<0.01)
Attempted suicide	All 1.00	(<0.72)
Divorced	All 1.00	(<0.78)
Loss of significant relationship	ICA 2.64	(<0.01)
Treatment for emotional problems	ICA 4.60	(<0.01)
	PT 5.00	(<0.01)
Unable to perform activities of a parent	ICA 1.28	(<0.01)
	PT 1.15	(<0.06)
Unable to perform other activities including sex, working, exercise, travel, pregnancy	ICA 2.64	(<0.01)

[a] Other covariates include, age, sex, education and sample. Results are relative to the GPOP (comparison) sample.
[b] Comparison sample GPOP.
[c] Probability of a type 1 statistical error, two sided; comparing IC samples with the GPOP sample.

with IC were five times as likely as the comparison sample to have been treated for emotional problems, and also more likely to be unable to perform the activities of being a parent.

Using well-developed quality of life indicators, which employed responses to subjective statements, Held et al. reported that IC females scored lower on nine such tests, compared with an identical set of tests given to a sample of US females with chronic renal failure undergoing dialysis. These tests, which are described in Campbell et al. (1976), were also used by Evans et al. (1981) in their study of patients with chronic renal disease. Three examples of these tests are shown in Fig. 4.2. In all cases the IC samples had worse scores and each of the separate samples were statistically different from the female dialysis patients.

Discussion

The medical literature contains numerous articles which tangentially relate to the nature of the epidemiology of interstitial cystitis. Collectively, these articles have provided an overview of many aspects of this disease which, viewed today with more definitive information, support some of the current beliefs and findings and contradict others. In fact, most of the previous literature, which may have accurately reflected the situation in one practice or clinic, could not

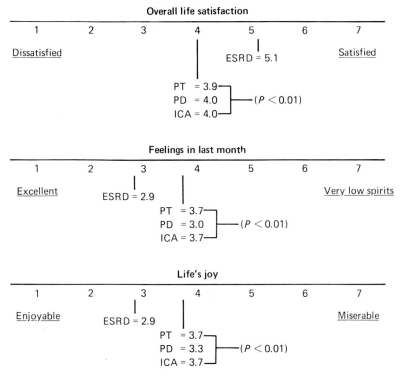

Fig. 4.2. Measures of quality of life in female end–stage renal disease patients (*ESRD*) and IC patients (*PT*, *PD*, and *ICA*, 1984–1987). Other tests were used with similar results. *P* value refers to the test between ESRD and the PT, PD, and ICA sample, separately. Questions are from Campbell et al. (1976).

properly be generalized to a larger universe given the case study basis of most of these reports.

One article in the literature does stand out because it contains a more definitive attempt to conduct a population-based analysis which justified more generalization to a larger universe. Oravisto's (1975) report stands as the definitive article on several aspects of IC but especially on incidence and prevalence. Oravisto's work suggests that if extrapolated to the USA, the prevalence (total number of cases) would be 22 000 females, with an incidence of 1400 new cases per year. Put differently, these estimates would imply that if all IC female patients were treated and diagnosed only by urologists, on average urologists would have less than three such females in their practice and would make one new diagnosis every 5 years! (In contrast, Held et al. estimated that, on average, board-certified urologists had 10 diagnosed IC females in their practice and 78% made at least one diagnosis in the previous year.) If one considers that at least some IC patients would see other specialists, the low frequency implied by the Oravisto estimates is only worsened. Adding male cases would not change the basic picture since practically all sources agree that this is primarily, but not totally, a female ailment.

Recent epidemiologic investigations by Held et al. (1989a, b, c) have contributed substantially to our knowledge of interstitial cystitis. Urologists of different ages, for example, appear to use the same criteria in diagnosing IC. But the work of Held et al. raises several issues that are not yet resolved and are of primary importance in determining the social priority of IC research. Held et al. estimate a *diagnosed* prevalence and incidence of IC in the USA that is approximately two to three times that implied by Oravisto. But even more importantly, Held et al. find that for every diagnosed case of IC there appear to be approximately four other cases that have strong resemblance to IC in that they have two of the classic symptoms, i.e., a painful bladder and sterile non-bacterial urine. The third criterion, which forms the basis of the current diagnostic specification, namely glomerulation with hydraulic distension under general anesthesia, cannot be confirmed or denied with the current data. Consequently, the implications of these painful bladder, sterile urine cases remain fundamentally important and of considerable interest.

While the Held et al. estimates of diagnosed prevalance and incidence of IC are substantially higher than the Oravisto estimates for Helsinki as extrapolated to the USA, the medical literature appears to be very accepting of the notion that the Oravisto estimates are likely to be biased low. Oravisto himself felt that his estimates were "minima" and that rates are "likely to have been rising in the more recent past." Numerous other authors since that time (e.g., Messing 1984; Meares 1987) have reported both that the published prevalence and incidence estimates are too low and that the rates are on the rise.

Clearly, future efforts at improving and confirming the estimates of incidence and prevalence are most desirable. Without more definitive information, there will be claims that may not have a scientific basis but which are used and quoted for a variety of reasons. For example, one source (American Foundation for Urologic Diseases 1980) cites an estimate of 450 000 cases of IC in the USA. This estimate is at the upper end of the range described by Held et al. (1987a) and is not their best midpoint estimate. The largest uncertainty in the Held et al. work is the classification of the potential but unconfirmed cases of IC (painful bladder and sterile urine). However, if one considers patients seen by other physician specialties and patients not in the medical care system at all, which one must, then even these counts may be biased low. There is a consensus that Oravisto's estimate is probably too low. But how much too low cannot be said with certainty.

Without totally resolving the conflict, can we reconcile these disparate findings of Oravisto and Held et al.? One possible explanation is that the definition of IC has been changing. This was suggested by Meares (1987) and others. For example, the work of Stamm and his colleagues (1982) opens the possibility that uretheral syndrome cases of the past might be diagnosed as IC in the current environment. In any case, the evidence presented here, as well as the popular literature and media, strongly suggest that the number of females with chronic non-bacterial painful bladder far exceeds any estimates based on the 1975 report of Oravisto.

Interstitial cystitis patients are almost always diagnosed by a urologist; 95% of the ICA sample reported such a source of diagnosis. While the time from onset to diagnosis is large by any standard (24 to 51 months on average), it is remarkably less than the 6–7 years reported by Oravisto (1975). Given the consistency of the responses to diagnostic criteria, by the board-certified urologists in the Held et al. study, one question to ponder is whether there is a problem in the system by which patients are referred to urologists. The lack of

IC diagnoses by nonurologists, and the significant number of nonurologists seen by IC patients en route to a diagnosis, suggests that other physicians may fail to diagnose and/or refer the IC patient to a urologist. While we do not know the specifics of Finland, the general perception is that in much of Europe it is more difficult for a patient to see a specialist than is the case in the USA. This possibility is certainly consistent with the long time to diagnosis in Finland. These hypotheses suggest that the issue of access and proper referral to specialists is one for future research.

One of the distinct changes in the medical communities' perception of IC is the age at onset. While the literature has generally alleged that IC can occur at almost any age, IC was historically viewed as primarily a post-menopause disease. The work by Held and colleagues clearly shows that the disease is more common in younger women than was previously believed. As shown in Fig. 4.1, in both the ICA sample and the PD sample over 25% of the diagnosed patients were less than 30 years of age at onset.

The work by Held et al. was based on three separate samples of diagnosed IC patients. One (ICA) was a self-selected sample of women with IC. The other two were patients recently treated (PT) and recently diagnosed (PD) by a random sample of urologists. While the efforts to keep these samples separate made the analysis complex, each of these samples made a separate contribution to the analysis. In many dimensions these three samples were similar but in some dimensions there were notable differences. The ICA sample is based on membership in a self-help and advocacy group and, as such, might be expected to represent more severe cases on average. Compared to the other patient samples, the ICA sample saw more physicians before a diagnosis was made, experienced a substantially longer period between onset and diagnosis, and have had IC for a longer time period.

The economic cost of treating IC is far from trivial. But because the patients are usually treated on an ambulatory basis, the cost per patient, while substantial, is less than some chronic diseases. As a result, the case for achieving medical cost reduction through research on prevention or cure is less strong than for more costly diseases. However, the cost of treatment is only part of the true cost to society. The loss of employment and the reduced wages for those who do work as well as the low quality of life are much larger costs than the direct medical costs.

When a society is choosing which medical research to fund, it is generally agreed that, other factors being equal, diseases that claim many victims should have higher priority than diseases with fewer victims, assuming that the severity of the illnesses are the same. So too with the severity of the impairment. In other words, the social damage caused by the disease is proportional to the number of patients affected and to the severity and length of the ailment. This is one of the reasons why better IC prevalence estimates would be helpful and why the job and quality of life loss resulting from IC are also relevant in measuring the social damage of this disease. Length of the social loss is proportional to the time a patient has the disease, which is why the younger age at onset is relevant.

Since medical research is a social investment, the social costs of the disease are only part of the equation; of equal importance is the likely cost of the cure, once discovered, including the cost of the research needed to find the cure. Consequently, a case can be made that when choosing among research projects, all other factors being equal, it is desirable to focus on those diseases whose treatment or cure is likely to be of lower cost. Since it is probable that the cure of IC is not likely to involve costly organ replacement such as a mechanical heart or other "high-tech" approaches, research into IC would fulfil these criteria.

One issue that has not received much attention in the IC literature is whether the cases of IC that are diagnosed and treated may be biased towards upper income and more highly educated Americans. For example, such a situation would be consistent with the notion that it takes above average determination and financial resources to contend with numerous physician visits that frequently end in little or no satisfaction for the patient. This situation might also be consistent with the low frequency of diagnosed IC for black Americans.

The evidence presented by Held et al. (1987a) suggests that this may be the case in the USA today. All three samples of IC patients (ICA, PT, PD) had above average income; however, given that they are younger on average than the control sample, the true difference may even be larger. (We assume here that higher income does not cause IC.) Two pieces of evidence do contradict this hypothesis of a relationship between social status and diagnosis of IC. First, the estimates from the PD sample showed that blacks were represented at the level of their numbers in the comparison sample, and, second, the education levels of the IC samples were equal to the comparison sample. While the family income of the PD sample was higher than that for the comparison sample, it was less than the income of the PT and ICA sample, i.e., the new patients more nearly represented the comparison sample while the PT patients (last treated) were definitely higher than the comparison sample. Like many other areas of research on IC, this is hardly a closed issue and further research is warranted.

Appendix: Screening Criteria

Table 4A.1. Screening criteria for future trials[a]

Interstitial cystitis patient accrual form

Automatic exclusions
<18 years of age
Benign or malignant bladder tumors
Radiation cystitis
Bacterial cystitis
Vaginitis
Cytoxan cystitis
Symptomatic urethral diverticulum
Uterine, cervical, vaginal, urethral carcinoma
Active herpes
Bladder calculi, lower ureteral calculi

Waking frequency <5X in 12 hours
Nocturia <2
Symptoms relieved by antibiotics, urinary antiseptics, urinary analgesics (e.g. pyridium)
Duration <12 months
Involuntary bladder contractions (urodynamics)
Capacity >400 ml, absence of sensory urgency

Table 4A.1. (Continued)

Interstitial cystitis patient accrual form

Automatic inclusions
Hunner's ulcer

Positive factors
Pain on bladder filling relieved by emptying
Pain – suprapubic, pelvic, urethral, vaginal, perineal
Glomerulations on endoscopy
Decreased compliance on cystometrogram

Bladder distension is arbitrarily defined as 80 cm water pressure for 1 min.
Two positive factors are necessary to be included in the study population.
Substratification at conclusion of study by bladder capacity under anesthesia: >350 ml, <350 ml.
[a] Adapted at the NIDDK Workshop on Interstitial Cystitis held in Bethesda, Maryland, on 28–29 August 1987.

References

American Foundation For Urologic Diseases (1980) Research progress and promises. American Foundation for Urologic Diseases, Baltimore

Bowers JE, Lattimer JK (1957) Interstitial cystitis. Surg Gynecol Obstet 105:313

Campbell A, Converse PE, Rodgers WL (1976) The quality of American life; perception, evaluations and satisfactions. Russell Sage Foundation, New York, pp 528, 554

Carson RB (1953) Management of vesicourethral dysfunction in women. JAMA 153:1152

De Juana CP, Everett JC (1977) Interstitial cystitis, experience and review of recent literature. Urology 10:325–329

Evans RW, Manninen DL, Garrison LP et al. (1981) Procedures manual for the national kidney dialysis and kidney transplantation study. Battelle Human Affairs Research Centers, Seattle

Farkas A, Waisman J, Goodwin WE (1977) Interstitial cystitis in adolescent girls. J Urol 118:837–839

Freiha FS, Faysal MH, Stamey TA (1980) The surgical treatment of intractable interstitial cystitis. J Urol 123:632–634

Geist RW, Antolak SJ Jr (1970) Interstitial cystitis in children. J Urol 104:922–925

Hand JR (1949) Interstitial cystitis: report of 223 cases (204 women and 19 men). J Urol 61:291–310

Hanno P, Wein A (1987) Interstitial cystitis, Parts I and II. American Urological Association, Baltimore. (Update series, lesson 9, vol 1)

Hanno PM, Wein AJ, Held PJ, Pauly MV, Cahn MA (1990) Diagnosis of interstitial cystitis. (Unpublished data)

Held PJ, Hanno PM, Wein AJ, Pauly MV, Cahn MA (1987a) Study of women with painful bladder syndrome. Presented at NIDDK Workshop on Interstitial Cystitis, Bethesda, Maryland, 28–29 August 1987

Held PJ, Pauly MV, Diamond L (1987b) Survival analysis of patients undergoing dialysis. JAMA 257(5):645–650

Held PJ, Hanno PM, Wein AJ, Pauly MV, Cahn MA (1990) Economic and social cost of interstitial cystitis

Held PJ, Hanno PM, Wein AJ, Pauly MV, Cahn MA (1990) Epidemiology of interstitial cystitis

Held PJ, Hanno PM, Wein AJ, Pauly MV, Cahn MA (1990) Prevalence and incidence of interstitial cystitis

Hunner GL (1915) A rare type of bladder ulcer in women; report of cases. Boston Med Surg J 172:660–664

Kinder CH, Smith RD (1958) Hunner's ulcer. Br J Urol 30:338–343

Lapides J (1975) Observations on interstitial cystitis. Urology 5:610·611

McDonald HP, Upchurch WE, Artime M (1958) Bladder dysfunction in children caused by interstitial cystitis. J Urol 80:354–356

Meares EM Jr (1987) Guest editorial. Interstitial cystitis – 1987. Urology (suppl) 29(4)

Messing EM (1984) Interstitial cystitis and related syndromes. In: Walsh PC, Gittes RF, Perlmutter AD, Stamey TA (eds) Campbell's urology, 5th edn. Saunders, Philadelphia

Messing EM (1987) Interstitial cystitis – 1987. Urology (suppl) 29(4)

Messing EM, Stamey TA (1978) Interstitial cystitis: early diagnosis, pathology, and treatment. Urology 12:381–392

Oravisto KJ (1975) Epidemiology of interstitial cystitis. Ann Chir Gynaecol Fenn 64:75–77

Oravisto KJ, Alfthan OS, Jokinen EJ (1970) Interstitial cystitis: clinical and immunological findings. Scand J Urol Nephrol 4:37–42

Parivar F, Bradbrook RA (1986) Interstitial cystitis. Br J Urol 58:239–244

Pool TL (1967) Interstitial cystitis: clinical considerations and treatment. Clin Obstet Gynecol 10:185–191

Roback G, Mead D, Randolph L (1986) Physician characteristics and distribution in the US, 1986 edition. American Medical Association, Chicago

Smith BH, Dehner LP (1972) Chronic ulcerating interstitial cystitis (Hunner's ulcer). Arch Pathol 93:76–81

Stamm WE, Counts GW, Running KR, Fihn S, Truck M, Holmes KK (1982) Diagnosis of coliform infection in acutely dysuric women. N Engl J Med 307(8):463–468

Statistical Abstract of the United States 1988, 108th edition. US Department of Commerce, Washington

Von Garrelts B (1966) Interstitial cystitis: thirteen patients treated operatively with intestinal bladder substitutes. Acta Chir Scand 132:436–443

Walsh A (1978) Interstitial cystitis. In: Harrison JH, Gittes RF, Perlmutter AD, Stamey TA, Walsh PC (eds) Campbell's Urology, 4th edn. Saunders, Philadelphia

Chapter 5

Interstitial Cystitis: Animal Models

M.R. Ruggieri, F.C. Monson, R.M. Levin, A.J. Wein and
P.M. Hanno

Introduction

There exists a very large group of patients with mundane sounding, but
sometimes disabling symptoms for which we have no explanation or rational
treatment. Interstitial cystitis (IC) is an example of a condition for which few
specific diagnostic criteria have been established, the diagnosis resting upon the
experience and personal bias of the physician. It is largely a diagnosis of
exclusion. A given collection of signs and symptoms which would form an
acceptable basis for the diagnosis in one clinic might not be considered
appropriate in another (Hald and Holm-Bentzen 1986).

Misconceptions abound in the literature and are partly responsible for the
hopeless attitude adopted by many patients, as the information is relayed
through their general physicians. An editorial in the *British Medical Journal*
stated that "all authorities agree that without treatment the condition is chronic
and progressive, without remissions or spontaneous cure" (Anon 1972).

Interstitial cystitis, as described by Walsh (1978) in *Campbell's Urology*, is "a
disease of extremes: extremely severe symptoms; extremes of underdiagnosis
and overdiagnosis; etiologic theories varying from the abstruse to the
fashionable; treatment ranging from the alpha of vitamin prescription to the
omega of radical bladder substitution surgery; and, sadly often, extreme
confusion in medical thinking." The true incidence of this condition in the
general population is not accurately known. Without uniform diagnostic criteria
to define the disease, it is impossible to compare prevalence data reported by
different investigators using different criteria. The only sizable epidemiologic
study was done in Helsinki, Finland, where the genetic homogeneity of the
population is perhaps not comparable with the rest of the human population.
The prevalence was reported to be 10.6 cases per 100 000, with the ratio of
women to men being slightly more than 10 to 1 (Oravisto 1975). The disease has
appeared more frequently in recent years, perhaps due to increased awareness
and recognition, and the greater care with which physicians diagnose and treat
lower urinary tract infections (Messing and Stamey 1978). Subjective
symptomatology includes a marked increased in urgency and frequency of

urination (which can be every 15 min) and lower abdominal pain (mild to severe). Only in its more advanced state (classic IC) are objective criteria utilized to diagnose the disease. These objective criteria include decreased bladder capacity, decreased compliance, atrophy of the musculature, petechia upon distension, and the appearance of "Hunner's ulcers" (Shipton 1965).

The presence of immunoreactive substances and mast cells is now the basis of the histopathologic diagnosis of IC. An autoimmune etiology was hypothesized as far back as 1938, when similarities between interstitial cystitis and lupus erythematosus (LE) were recognized (Fister 1938). Since then there has been a steady stream of reports describing different immunological abnormalities of IC patients. None of these investigations have identified any single immunopathology consistently present in all or even most IC patients studied (Oravisto et al. 1970; Silk 1970; Jokinen et al. 1972a, b, 1973; Gordon et al. 1973; Boye et al. 1979; de la Serna and Alarcon-Sefovia 1981; Weisman et al. 1981; Mattila 1982, Mattila et al. 1983; Lose et al. 1983). Numerous investigators have reported increased mast cells in the muscularis (Simmons and Bruce 1958; Sissons 1961; Bohne et al. 1962; Silk 1970; Collan et al. 1976; de Juana and Everett 1977; Larsen et al. 1982; Kastrup et al. 1983), prompting one group to suggest that a more appropriate name for the condition might be "detrusor mastocytosis" (Larsen et al. 1982). When examined with the electron microscope, the mast cells in the bladder of IC patients were observed to be partially or completely degranulated, whereas this was not found in any of the control tissues (Collan et al. 1976; Larsen et al. 1982). Adenosine triphosphate (ATP), the molecule most cells employ to store intracellular energy, is known to initiate noncytotoxic degranulation of mast cell suspensions (Keller 1966). The potential importance of ATP-induced mast cell degranulation is the observation that ATP or a related compound may be the neurotransmitter responsible for the nonadrenergic, noncholinergic (possibly purinergic) contractions of the urinary bladder (Burnstock 1972). A purinergic neurotransmitter discharged from purinergic nerves in the vicinity of mast cells may induce degranulation and thus liberation of histamine (Riley and West 1953) from the mast cell granules. This histamine from the mast cells together with the purinergic neurotransmitter may then cause contraction of the bladder smooth muscle (Khanna et al. 1977). Indirect evidence for this has been presented by Sjogren and associates who found that in vitro bladder strips from patients with prostatic hypertrophy and "unstable bladders" (IC?) were more resistant to atropine inhibition of electrically induced contractions (Sjogren et al. 1982).

The etiology is unknown but it is not generally thought to be associated with bacterial or viral infection (with the possible exception of proviral forms or slow-growing viruses). Even this is somewhat controversial in view of the very recent demonstration of *Chlamydia* in some patients (Bruce et al. 1985). The failure to find an infectious agent certainly does not constitute proof of a noninfectious etiology since the vector may not be easily cultured or otherwise detected in the laboratory. Indeed, the immunological findings, which have been given a great deal of attention in the past, may be secondary to a covert infectious etiology. Nevertheless, an infectious theory of etiology for IC has virtually been abandoned (Hanno and Wein 1987).

Several groups have theorized that the condition may be related to a primary defect in the bladder mucin glycosaminoglycan (GAG) layer. The substances of the glycosaminoglycan class which are of primary importance are hyaluronic acid, heparin sulfate, heparin, chondroitin 4-sulfate, chondroitin 6-sulfate, dermatan sulfate and keratin sulfate. These carbohydrate chains, coupled to protein cores, are known as the proteoglycans, which are probably among the most important and least studied of all the biological macromolecules (Trelstad 1985). Parsons proposed that IC might be caused by a deficiency in the bladder surface mucin layer, suggesting treatment with synthetic GAG (Parsons et al. 1983). There are indications that in elderly subjects the urothelium may be prone to increased leakage, leaving the bladder tissue more exposed to urine-borne chemicals and carcinogens (Jacob et al. 1978). It has been proposed that suppression of the water-tight nature of the normal bladder could be at the origin of the disease, with the possibility of infiltration of urine into the bladder wall (Lepinard et al. 1984).

An ultrastructural study reported by Collan and coworkers in 1976 on the bladder epithelium found only similarities between IC patients and controls (Collan et al. 1976). In a more recent study, Dixon et al. (1986) concluded that there are absolutely no differences in the morphologic appearances of the glycocalyx or urothelial cells in patients with IC when compared with controls. In a previous study (Eldrup et al. 1983), the possibility was raised that an increase in the permeability of the urothelium might be an etiologic factor in IC by demonstrating that, in contrast to controls, colloidal lanthanum penetrated between the surface urothelial cells in some patients. Leakage of the urothelium was attributed to defective tight junctions between adjacent urothelial cells. Dixon's study, however, showed that penetration of ruthenium red between surface urothelial cells occurred similarly in samples from both IC patients and controls. Hence, the hypothesis that an important pathogenic factor in IC is a defective glycocalyx associated with a permeable urothelium has not been supported. Using lectin binding histochemistry, Sant looked for alterations in bladder GAGs in IC patients and found that many of the carbohydrate terminals of bladder surface GAGs are unchanged in the disease. An increased incidence of galactose and fucose terminals, of questionable significance, was noted in some patients (Sant et al. 1986).

The knowledge that substances in the urine can penetrate an intact bladder mucosa into the deeper layers, while not a specific finding for IC, has opened a new avenue for research into its etiology – the possibility that agents in the urine peculiar to patients with IC may initiate the pathologic process in the bladder leading to the illness. Dr. Edward M. Messing, Associate Professor of Urology, University of Wisconsin, in an unpublished observation (personal communication), reported the presence of a substance in the urine of patients with confirmed IC that will contract isolated smooth muscle strips. This myogenic substance was not present in the urine of either normal subjects or patients without IC. This might be consistent with the release of histamine (or other myogenic substances) within the wall of the bladder with the subsequent diffusion into the bladder mucosa and secretion into the urine.

Current Research Strategies

Of the several possible etiologies presented, we have directed our initial attention to the relationship between IC and the properties of the surface of the bladder lumen. There is a large body of evidence which demonstrates that the mucosal surface of the urinary bladder is important in both inhibiting the ability of microorganisms to colonize the bladder urothelium and protecting the bladder from substances excreted in the urine.

Experimental Models

Mucin-deficient Rabbit Bladder Model (see Hanno et al. 1978, 1983; Ruggieri et al. 1984)

Bacterial adherence to the urinary bladder is assayed as follows: male New Zealand white rabbits weighing 2–2.5 kg are anesthetized with 1.5 ml ketamine/ xylazine (7 : 5 v/v) i.m. supplemented with nembutal (50 mg/ml) i.v. to effect. Rabbits are secured, the urinary bladders catheterized with a #8 French catheter and the bladders emptied. Prior to introduction of ^{3}H-labeled bacteria the bladders are flushed three times with 10 ml aliquots of saline introduced through the catheter. For mucin-deficient model, a 1 min, 10 ml, 50% acetone bladder wash is performed prior to the three saline washes described above. Approximately 8×10^8 CFU labeled bacteria in 1.5 ml is introduced through the catheter and flushed in with 5 ml of saline. After 20 min exposure to the labeled bacteria the bladders are flushed three times with 10 ml aliquots of saline. The animal is then sacrificed with i.v. T-61 Euthanasia solution (Hoechst Corp.), the bladder removed and the mucosa dissected free from the underlying muscle layer and assayed for ^{3}H activity.

The effect of heparin or other agents on bacterial adherence is determined by washing the bladder with 10 ml of the agent (1 min) prior to the three 10 ml saline washes as described above. In testing these agents in the mucin-deficient bladder model, the agent is added after the mucin is extracted.

Bacterial Adherence to Anion Exchange Resin (see Hanno et al. 1984; Ruggieri et al. 1985, 1986)

The ability of chemical agents and bladder mucosal extracts to prevent bacterial adherence to anion exchange resin is assayed in vitro as follows: A strong anion exchange resin (AG1-X2, 200–400 mesh, Bio-Rad, Rockville Center, New York) with quaternary ammonium ion as the active group is gently swirled in 50 mM, pH 7.0 buffer (tris (hydroxymethyl)-aminomethane hydrochloride), decanted four times to remove fines and suspended at 50% settled bed volume. The resin slurrys are made up weekly and stored at 2–4 °C between experiments.

For the adherence assays the resin slurry is gently swirled and 0.8 ml is quickly pipetted into 13×100 mm test tubes. To the resin is added 1 ml of buffer or serial dilutions of various chemical agents or bladder extracts in buffer, and 200 µl of radiolabeled bacterial. The resin–bacteria mixture is incubated at 27 °C for 10 min. At the end of the incubation, 5 ml of buffer is added to the tubes, and the resin with attached bacteria is filtered using 10µm pore size Teflon filters (Millipore LCWP 02500) to retain the resin with attached bacteria while allowing unattached organisms to pass through. The resin is then washed four times with 5 ml aliquots of buffer, scraped off of the filter and placed in 7 ml scintillation vials; 6 ml of Hydrofluor scintillation fluid is added and the vials are vortexed. Radioactivity in counts per minute is determined in a Packard B2450 liquid scintillation spectrophotometer to generate bacterial adherence inhibition curves for each mucin sample.

Mucin Extraction

Rabbit Mucin (see Ruggieri et al 1985)

In catheterized rabbits, the bladder mucins are extracted with 10 ml washes of 50% acetone in H_2O. The acetone washes are combined, centrifuged at 1000g for 30 min and the precipitate discarded. The acetone is evaporated from the sample under mild heat and vacuum. The sample is then dialyzed overnight in deionized distilled H_2O. The aqueous mucin fraction is freeze-dried to a powder, weighed and stored in a desiccator at $-4\,°C$. The lyophylized mucin is dissolved at a concentration of 4 mg/ml in 50 mM tris buffer, pH 7.0 and serially diluted six times 1:2 in buffer for inhibition of bacterial adherence to anion exchange resin as described above.

Human Mucin

In catheterized patients, the urine is removed and the bladder washed with 100 ml of saline for 1 min. The saline is removed, dialyzed against distilled water overnight, and lyophylized to a powder.

Studies

The first line of defense against invading microorganisms in the urinary tract is the antiadherence activity of the surface mucin layer. Removing this mucin with 50% acetone increases bacterial adherence to the bladder mucosa by over 100-fold. Replacing the extracted mucin with either heparin or reconstituted mucin reduces bacterial adherence to the mucosa to control levels, as shown in Fig. 5.1 (Hanno et al. 1978, 1983; Ruggieri et al. 1984).

Our studies have demonstrated that bacterial adherence to anion exchange resin can be used as a model of adherence for the mucin-deficient rabbit bladder. Figure 5.2 demonstrates that agents which inhibit adherence to anion exchange resin also inhibit adherence to the mucin-deficient rabbit bladder (Hanno et al. 1984; Ruggieri et al. 1985, 1986). Figure 5.3 shows that dialyzed, lyophylized, saline extracts of bladder mucosa from several species, including man, also inhibit bacterial adherence to both the animal model and anion exchange resin (Ruggieri et al. 1985). The resin assay has an advantage over other methods of quantitation or visualization of mucin because it measures the capacity of a mucin sample to prevent bacterial adherence and does not merely determine the quantity of mucin. This is of extreme importance since it is this property of

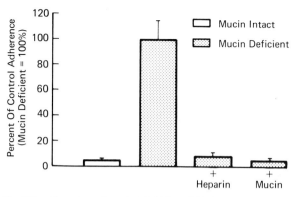

Fig. 5.1. Heparin and mucin inhibition of *Escherichia coli* adherence to the rabbit urinary bladder.

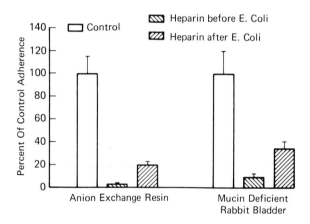

Fig. 5.2. Heparin inhibition and displacement of *E. coli* adherence.

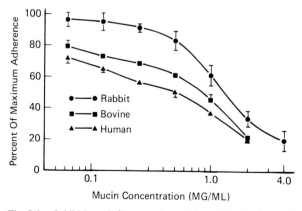

Fig. 5.3. Inhibition of adherence to resin by rabbit, bovine and human bladder extracts.

mucin that is believed to protect the bladder from not only bacterial colonization but also from the irritative effects of substances in urine.

Using this method of analysis, a study has been performed which demonstrates that mucin derived from patients with recurrent urinary tract infections is less potent at inhibiting bacterial adherence to anion exchange resin than mucin derived from IC and other groups of patients.

Specifically, four groups of patients were studied. Two groups of pediatric patients (10 patients in each group) were from Cardinal Glennon Children's hospital in St. Louis. These bladder extracts were collected by Dr. George F. Steinhardt, Assistant Professor of Pediatric Urology, St. Louis University School of Medicine. One of these groups consisted of patients with histories of frequent urinary tract infections (UTI) without any known specific etiology. The second group of pediatric patients had neurogenic bladders resulting from meningomyelocele requiring clean intermittent catheterization (CIC). This group of patients frequently had positive urinary tract cultures of $>10^5$ organisms per ml urine, presumably due to the catheterizations. The third group of 10 patients was diagnosed as having IC at the Women's Center for the Evaluation and Treatment of Interstitial Cystitis at the University of Pennysylvania (IC). The fourth group of patients (n=28) were from the Hospital of the University of Pennsylvania, where they were undergoing urodynamic evaluation for a variety of disorders including bladder outlet obstruction, incontinence, frequency/urgency symptoms, etc. (NONUTI).

A bar graph representing the data for inhibition of bacterial adherence to anion exchange resin by bladder extracts from the four groups is displayed in Fig. 5.4. As can be seen, the data for the UTI patients show that mucin from those bladders was much less capable of inhibiting bacterial adhesion than were bladder extracts from the other three groups, including the IC group.

These results represent the first demonstration of a defective antiadherence activity of bladder extracts (mucin) from patients with recurrent urinary tract infection. Most of the patients in this group (UTI) did have infections at the time of specimen collection; however, so did many of the other pediatric patients (CIC). Thus, the mere presence of urinary tract infection cannot be the cause of the defective mucin in the UTI group. The bladder extracts from the IC group

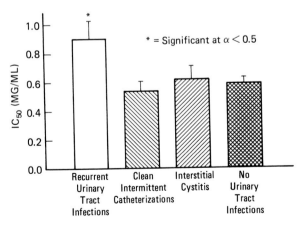

Fig. 5.4. Potency of human bladder extracts to inhibit bacterial adherence to resin.

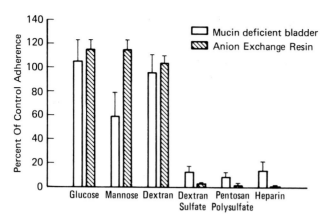

Fig. 5.5. Effect of various agents on *E. coli* adherence to the bladder and resin.

showed antiadherence activity identical to the CIC and NONUTI group. This would indicate that the functional antiadherence activity of bladder mucin in IC is intact. Although there may be subtle differences in the mucin layer, its functional activity in terms of antibacterial adherence is identical in all patients studied except the UTI group. Although the amount of mucin recovered was mildly elevated in the UTI group, the effectiveness of the mucin to prevent bacterial adherence was reduced. Thus there may be a functional defect and/or decrease in a factor in the mucin that is responsible for increased bacterial adherence and increased incidence of infection in this group of patients. We are currently using the resin binding methodology to isolate the active component in mucin (Fig. 5.5).

Interstitial cystitis has received a considerable amount of publicity in the past few years in both lay publications and the television news media. One factor which has been circumstantially implicated in its etiology is prior antibiotic therapy (Gillespi et al. 1985). Although true IC has not been reported as a side effect of nitrofurantoin, tetracyline, sulfamethoxazole/trimethoprim or any other therapy in any peer-reviewed scientific publication, an abstract presented at the Western Regional American Urological Association (AUA) meeting and again by the same workers at the annual AUA meeting in Atlanta in 1985 has implicated several antibiotics as inducers of IC (Gillespi et al. 1985).

This evidence is based on the observation that many of the patients being diagnosed as having IC have been previously treated with antibiotics. This is not unusual considering that most of these women probably have had symptoms of cystitis for many years and therefore were at one time or another empirically treated with antibiotics based on their symptomatology. This abstract also claims that nitrofurantoin acts as a surface active agent (surfactant) that destroys glycosaminoglycan on the surface of the bladder when used even for very short time periods in the absence of infection.

In an attempt to use chronic antibiotic administration to create an animal model of interstitial cystitis, we studied both the acute and chronic effect of nitrofurantoin on the urinary bladder of rabbits:

Acute Administration of Nitrofurantoin

Acute studies were performed to discover the effects of nitrofurantoin (at more than double the normal therapeutic concentration) on the periodic acid-Schiff (PAS) staining, structural integrity of the bladder luminal surface, and on bacterial adherence (Ruggieri et al. 1987). For comparative purposes, a true surfactant (Triton X-100) and organic solvents were also tested.

The most important result of this investigation was that exposure of the bladder to 1.0 mM nitrofurantoin for 1 min did not remove the mucin layer nor increase bacterial adherence. (1.0 mM nitrofurantoin is the highest concentration possible for this agent in water because of its limited solubility.) This is at least twice the urinary concentrations found 0–24 h following a therapeutic dose of 100 mg q.i.d. (Lippman et al. 1958). One must conclude from this result that nitrofurantoin does not remove or destroy the functional integrity of the bladder luminal surface mucin layer as has been suggested by other workers (Gillespi et al. 1985). While the time of exposure in this preliminary study was brief, the drug concentration presented to the bladder was over twice as high as that used in normal clinical situations. The sensitivity of the adherence assay would be expected to show any significant negative effect on the bladder surface. A similar exposure of the bladder mucosa to an equimolar concentration of the true surfactant Triton X-100 caused a greater than eightfold increase in bacterial adherence.

Fifty per cent dimethyl sulfoxide (DMSO) was also used in this investigation since it is used intravesically in the treatment of IC (Anon 1972; Messing and Stamey 1978; Walsh 1978; Hanno and Wein 1987). It is reassuring to know that this therapeutic agent does not impair the antiadherence capacity of the bladder epithelium. Other organic solvents (hexane, 50% acetone and 50% ethanol) did increase bacterial adherence to the bladder. One could interpret this result as indicating that the antiadherence factor of the bladder luminal surface is not very soluble in DMSO, whereas it is readily soluble in hexane, 50% acetone or 50% ethanol (see Fig. 5.6).

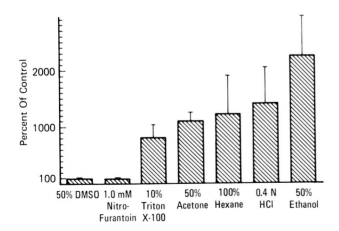

Fig. 5.6. Effect of various agents on bacterial adherence to the bladder.

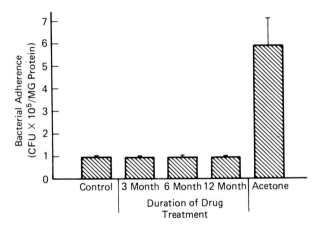

Chronic Administration of Nitrofurantoin

A second study (Levin et al. 1988) was conceived to investigate the chronic effects of antibiotic therapy using assays for in vivo bacterial adherence and in vitro mucin antiadherence activity combined with light microscopic and ultrastructural morphologic studies. Nitrofurantoin was chosen for these studies based on the extensive use of this agent in the treatment of urinary tract infection and the specific reference to this agent in the etiology of IC. This study has demonstrated that up to 1 year of chronic nitrofurantoin therapy induces no changes in the bacterial adherence characteristics of the rabbit bladder mucosa, specific antibacterial adherence activity of the bladder mucin, or ultrastructure of the mucosal layer, epithelial layer, interstitium, or muscularis.

Figure 5.7 displays the bacterial adherence of the control, and of animals treated for 3, 6 and 12 months with nitrofurantoin, as well as the effect of acetone for comparison. These results demonstrate that chronic nitrofurantoin

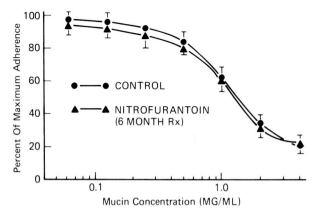

Fig. 5.8.   Inhibition of bacterial adherence by bladder mucin extract.

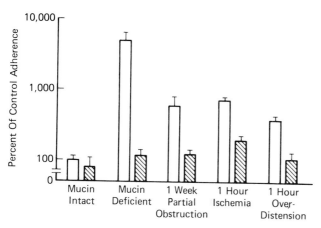

Fig. 5.9. Effect of experimental in vivo pathology on bacterial adherence.

administration for 12 months does not affect bacterial adherence to the in vivo rabbit bladder. Figure 5.8 shows that after 6 months of chronic treatment with nitrofurantoin the antiadherence activity of the bladder mucin is essentially identical to that of control animals.

Although chronic nitrofurantoin did not alter bacterial adherence of bladder mucin, other experimental models have been shown to result in markedly increased bacterial adherence to bladder mucosa. Figure 5.9 compares the bacterial adherence capacities of bladders which have been subjected to chemical stripping (mucin deficient), 1 week partial outlet obstruction, 1 h in vivo ischemia and 1 h acute overdistension. In addition, the ameliorative effect of a GAG component heparin was also tested. It is apparent that these induced pathologies cause significant decreases in antiadherence characteristics of the bladder mucosa. Whether these perturbations are transient or not remains the subject of further investigation.

What Constitutes an Experimental Animal Model of Interstitial Cystitis?

The above studies, with exceptions as noted, have been carried out using animals whose urinary tracts facilitate experimentation on one or more of the symptoms which comprise the symptomatic complex called Interstitial Cystitis. The complicated array of symptoms causes confusion in both diagnosis and study. To study this disease in humans is to impose a tremendous responsibility on the investigator to collect data on the full range of symptoms normally associated with it. Such a mass of data can only be reasonably collected with computer and data base assistance. Analysis surely will require the aid of computer-based statistical packages and cannot, at this point, be reasonably expected to provide definitive information and solutions to the problems of treatment.

Further, on the experimental level, it is clear that to design and implement experiments which involve patients requires consideration of cost, timing and controls. There are experiments which can be performed on human groups which can reasonably be expected to yield valuable information on IC, but the evidence thus far suggests that insufficient information exists at present to permit design and implementation of true problem solving experiments on human subjects.

A novel approach to the development of animal models to investigate complex problems is described by Desrosiers and Letvin in a recent paper on AIDS. They have quite satisfactorily approached the question of how to deal with the problem of future AIDS research. They state that, "An ideal [animal] model for AIDS would be one in which HIV infects and induces an AIDS-like disease in a readily available laboratory animal." They suggest that in the absence of such a suitable model, the most productive strategy is to partition the symptoms of AIDS such that suitable animal models for each symptom to be developed with the idea that an etiologic solution for each symptom will be facilitated by such compartmentalization of effort (Desrosiers and Letvin 1987).

Having in mind the fact that IC does not have a definite etiologic cause, we would suggest that the use of animal models to study isolated symptoms of IC will assist and greatly speed the process of investigation. Indeed, it is clear that if one takes this approach, much of the information available from urodynamic, physiologic, pharmacologic and anatomic literature on urinary bladders of human and various laboratory animals provides a foundation on which such a research effort can be based. A compartmentalized approach to the study of the symptoms of IC can best be initiated by utilizing extant and well-documented animal models as well as appropriate new models (e.g., an animal model for detrusor mastocytosis or an induced bladder hypersensitivity model). If conducted in this manner, there is much greater probability that basic investigations on the etiologies of the components of the IC symptom complex will yield clues to the root cause(s) of IC.

References

Anon (1972) Interstitial cystitis. Br Med J i:644–645

Bohne AW, Hodson JM, Rebuck JW, Reinhard RE (1962) An abnormal leukocyte response in interstitial cystitis. J Urol 88(3):387–391

Boye E, Morse M, Hutter I, Erlanger BF, MacKinnon KJ, Klassen J (1979) Immune complex – mediated interstitial cystitis as a major manifestation of systemic lupus erythematosus. Clin Immunol Immunopathol 13:67–76

Bruce AW, Reid G, Wong-Ho M, Duffy P, Drutz H, Costerton JW (1985) The role of chlamydia trachomatis in genito-urinary infections. J Urol 133(4):209A

Burnstock G (1972) Purinergic nerves. Pharmacol Rev 24:509–581

Collan Y, Alfthan O, Kivilaakso E, Oravisto KJ (1976) Electron microscopic and histological findings on urinary bladder epithelium in interstitial cystitis. Eur Urol 2:242–247

de Juana CP, Everett JC (1977) Interstitial cystitis. Experience and review of recent literature. Urology 10(4):325–329

de la Serna AR, Alarcon-Sefovia D (1981) Chronic interstitial cystitis as an initial major manifestation of systemic lupus erythematosus. J Rheumatol 8(5):808–810

Desrosiers RC, Letvin NL (1987) Animal models for acquired immunodeficiency syndrome. Rev Infect Dis 9(3):438–446

Dixon JS, Holm-Bentzen M, Gilpin CJ, Goslin JA, Bostofte E, Hald T, Larson S (1986) Electron microscopic investigation of the bladder urothelium and glycocalyx in patients with interstitial cystitis. J Urol 135:621–625

Eldrup J, Thorp J, Nielsen SL, Hald T, Hainau B (1983) Permeability and ultrastructure of human bladder epithelium. Br J Urol 55:488–492

Fister GM (1938) Similarity of interstitial cystitis (Hunner Ulcer) to lupus erythematosus. J Urol 40:37–51

Gillespi L, Said J, Cain W, Van der Veld R (1935) Antibiotic-induced interstitial cystitis: A model for cell membrane instability. J Urol 133(4):177A

Gordon HL, Rossen RD, Hirsh EM, Yium JJ (1973) Immunological aspects of interstitial cystitis. J Urol 109:228–233

Hald T, Holm-Bentzen M (1986) Clinical symptom complex. In: George NJR, Gosling JA (eds) Sensory disorders in the bladder and urethra. Springer, Berlin Heidelberg New York Tokyo, pp 49–62

Hanno PM, Wein AJ (1987) Interstitial cystitis, Parts 1 and 2. American Urological Association, Baltimore (AUA update series, volume 6, lesson 9 and 10)

Hanno PM, Fritz R, Wein AJ, Mulholland SG (1978) Heparin as antibacterial agent in rabbit bladder. Urology 12:411–416

Hanno PM, Ruggieri MR, Levin RM (1983) Adherence of several urinary tract pathogens: effects of heparin. Surg Forum 34:698–701

Hanno PM, Ruggieri MR, Levin RM (1984) Comparison of *Escherichia coli* adherence to the urinary bladder mucosa with adherence to anion exchange resin. Surg Forum 35:637–639

Jacob J, Ludgate CM, Forde J, Tulloch WS (1978) Recent observations on the ultrastructure of the human urothelium. Cell Tissue Res 193:543–560

Jokinen EJ, Lassen PA, Salo OP, Alfthan O (1972a) Discoid lupus erythematosus and interstitial cystitis. Ann Clin Res 4:23–25

Jokinen EJ, Alfthan OS, Oravisto KJ (1972b) Antitissue antibodies in interstitial cystitis. Clin Exp Immunol 11:333–339

Jokinen EJ, Oravisto KJ, Alfthan OS (1973) The effect of cystectomy on antitissue antibodies in interstitial cystitis. Clin Exp Immunol 15:457–460

Kastrup J, Hald T, Larsen S, Nielsen VG (1983) Histamine content and mast cell count of detrusor muscle in patients with interstitial cystitis and other types of chronic cystitis. Br J Urol 55:495–500

Keller R (1966) Tissue and mast cells in immune reactions Monogr Allergy 2:1–39

Khanna OP, DeGregorio GJ, Sample RG, McMichael RF (1977) Histamine receptors in urethrovesical smooth muscle. Urology 10(4):375–381

Larsen S, Thompson SA, Hald T, Barnard RJ, Gilpin CJ, Dixon JS, Gosling JA (1982) Mast cells in interstitial cystitis. Br J Urol 54:283–286

Lepinard V, Saint-Andre JP, Rogon LM (1984) La cystite interstitielle. J Urol (Paris) 90:455–465

Levin RM, Ruggieri MR, Lavkar RL, Hanno PM, Wein AJ (1982) Effect of chronic nitrofurantoin on the urinary bladder. J Urol 139:400–404

Lippman RW, Wrobel CJ, Ress R, Hoyt R (1958) A theory concerning recurrence of urinary infection: prolonged administration of nitrofurantoin for prevention. J Urol 80:77–81

Lose G, Frandsen B, Hojemsgard JC, Jespersen J, Astrup T (1983) Chronic interstitial cystitis: increased levels of eosinophil cationic protein in serum and urine and an ameliorating effect of subcutaneous heparin. Scand J Urol Nephrol 17:159–161

Mattila J (1982) Vascular immunopathy in interstitial cystitis. Clin Immunol Immunopathol 23:648–655

Mattila J, Harmoinen A, Hallstrom O (1983) Serum immunoglobulin and complement alterations in interstitial cystitis. Eur Urol 9:350–352

Messing EM, Stamey TS (1978) Interstitial cystitis. Early diagnosis, pathology and treatment. Urology 12(4):381–392

Oravisto KJ (1975) Epidemiology of interstitial cystitis. Ann Chir Gynaecol Fenn 64:75–77

Oravisto KJ, Alfthan OS, Jokinen EJ (1970) Interstitial cystitis. Clinical and immunological findings. Scand J Urol Nephrol 4:37–42

Parsons CL, Schmidt JD, Pollen JJ (1983) Successful treatment of interstitial cystitis with sodium pentosanpolysulfate. J Urol 130:51–53

Riley JF, West GB (1953) The presence of histamines in tissue mast cells. J Physiol (London) 120:528–537

Ruggieri MR, Hanno PM, Levin RM (1984) The effects of heparin on the adherence of five species of urinary tract pathogens to urinary bladder mucosa. Urol Res 12:199–203

Ruggieri MR, Hanno PM, Levin RM (1985) Further characterization of bacterial adherence to urinary bladder mucosa: comparison with adherence to anion exchange resin. J Urol 134:1019–1023

Ruggieri MR, Hanno PM, Levin RM (1986) Escherichia coli adherence to anion exchange resin: in vitro model for initial screening of potential antiadherence agents. Urology 28:343–348

Ruggieri MR, Hanno PM, Levin RM (1987) Nitrofurantoin is not a surface active agent in the rabbit urinary bladder. Urology 29:534–537

Sant GR, Ucci AA, Alroy J (1986) Bladder surface glycosaminoglycans in interstitial cystitis. J Urol 135:175A

Shipton EA (1965) Hunner's ulcer (chronic interstitial cystitis). A manifestation of collagen disease. Br J Urol 37:88–93

Silk MR (1970) Bladder antibodies in interstitial cystitis. J Urol 103:307–309

Simmons JL, Bruce PL (1958) On the use of an antihistamine in the treatment of interstitial cystitis. Am Surg 24:664–667

Sissons JL (1961) Interstitial cystitis: an explanation for the beneficial effect of an antihistamine. J Urol 85(2):149–155

Sjogren C, Andersson KE, Husted S, Mattiasson A, Moller-Madsen B (1982) Atropine resistance of transmurally stimulated isolated human bladder muscle. J Urol 128:1368–1371

Trelstad RL (1985) Glycosaminoglycans: mortar, matrix, mentor. Lab Invest 53:1–4

Walsh A (1978) Interstitial cystitis. In: Harrison JH, Gitter RF, Perlmutter AD, Stamey TA, Walsh PC (eds) Campbell's urology, 4th edn. Saunders, Philadelphia pp 693–707

Weisman MH, McDonald EC, Wilson CB (1981) Studies of the pathogenesis of interstitial cystitis, obstructive uropathy, and intestinal malabsorption in a patient with systemic lupus erythematosus. Am J Med 70:875–881

Chapter 6

Etiology: Etiologic and Pathogenetic Theories in Interstitial Cystitis

M. Holm-Bentzen, J. Nordling and T. Hald

Introduction

Painful bladder disease including interstitial cystitis is a symptom complex, first introduced by Borque (Borque 1951). There are painful bladder diseases with a known and an unknown etiology (Holm-Bentzen and Lose 1987; Holm-Bentzen et al. 1987c). All the patients present with a variety of urologic symptoms all of a more or less chronic nature: supra-retropubic pain, frequency, nocturia, urgency, dysuria and occasionally hematuria and stranguria (Hald and Holm-Bentzen 1986). The painful bladder diseases of a more specific nature and with a known etiology are listed in Table 6.1.

The painful bladder diseases of unknown etiology and pathogenesis are more difficult to define and describe precisely. Few specific diagnostic criteria are established, and the diagnoses rest upon the experience and personal bias of the physician or the urologist. It might be a diagnosis of exclusion. In the past few years our group has chosen to classify pathoanatomically the painful bladder diseases of unknown etiology (Holm-Bentzen 1985; Holm-Bentzen et al. 1987c). A thorough microscopic evaluation of a deep bladder biopsy in these patients

Table 6.1. The painful bladder diseases of a more specific nature

Irradiation cystitis
Cyclophosphamide cystitis
Cystitis caused by specific microorganisms
(chlamydia, TB, syphilis etc.)
Carcinoma in situ
Bladder cancer
Malacoplakia
Leukaemia
Systemic diseases (collagenosis, sarcoidosis)

can lead to a classification. We consider the following pathoanatomical diagnoses in these patients (Holm-Bentzen and Lose 1987):

1. Interstitial cystitis (Larsen et al. 1982)
2. Chronic unspecific cystitis
3. Detrusor myopathy (Holm-Bentzen et al. 1985)
4. Eosinophilic cystitis (Hellstrom et al. 1979)

Interstitial cystitis is defined pathoanatomically by an elevated mast cell count in the detrusor muscle, namely more than 28 mast cells/mm^2 (Larsen et al. 1982; Kastrup et al. 1983). Other studies have confirmed this (Lynes et al. 1986; Feltis et al. 1985), but there is still doubt as to whether an elevated number of mast cells also exist in the lamina propria (Larsen et al. 1982; Deane et al. 1983; Feltis et al. 1985; Lynes et al. 1986). Recently it has been reported that mast cells might even be present in the urothelium (Aldenborg et al. 1986).

The exact cause for the pathoanatomic findings in these patients are unknown. In the following we will focus on etiologic and pathogenetic theories concerning interstitial cystitis (IC) and try to rule out the most recent ones. We define IC as follows:

1. Chronic cystitis symptoms, including suprapubic pain, for at least one year
2. Sterile and cytologically normal urine
3. Most often, but not necessarily, an abnormal cystoscopy either before distension or petechial bleeding after distension
4. An elevated mast cell count in the detrusor muscle

No one knows whether this definition is right or wrong and in the literature other definitions have been used making comparisons between different studies difficult. The misconceptions in the literature are also partly responsible for the attitude of hopelessness that one sees in many patients after repeated visits to different physicians and urologists (Wein 1985).

General Remarks on Etiology and Pathogenesis

Many theories exist concerning etiology and pathogenesis in IC and these were reviewed recently by Messing (1986). The theories include infection, toxic agents in the urine, genetic or endocrinologic deficiencies, lymphatic or vascular obstruction, neurogenic, allergic or immune causes or defects in the cytoprotection of the bladder or even a psychiatric disease (Table 6.2).

Today, the general opinion is that the etiology is multifactorial, that the disease is caused by multiple factors and mechanisms and that we are dealing with a syndrome rather than a specific disease (Holm-Bentzen and Lose 1987).

The most predominant theories today are illustrated in Fig. 6.1. A substance in the urine, either a substance occurring in normal urine (a food-stuff, a metabolite, etc.) and only harmful to particularly susceptible bladders, or a substance not occurring in normal urine (a toxic agent), gains access to the bladder wall. This happens either through a defective glycosaminoglycans layer (GAG layer) or by destruction of a normal GAG layer, implying an easier

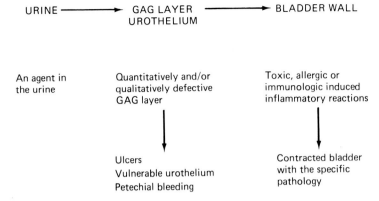

Fig. 6.1. Theories on the etiology and pathogenesis of interstitial cystitis.

penetration of the urothelium, since the natural cytoprotection of the bladder is impaired. The urothelium itself might be abnormally leaky. In the bladder wall inflammatory changes are included in IC implying mast cell degranulation, either toxically, allergically or immunologically. These changes might also be induced by a blood-borne agent, but it is reasonable to believe that urine plays a role, since patients with urinary diversions are relieved of their bladder symptoms (Linder and Smith 1958).

Table 6.2. Theories on the etiology and pathogenesis of interstitial cystitis

Infection
Extravesical foci of infection
Allergic, immune or autoimmune disorders
Defective cytoprotection
Toxic agents in urine
Genetic deficiencies
Endocrinological disturbances
Lymphatic obstruction
Vascular obstruction
Neurogenic disturbances
Psychiatric disease

The Etiologic Agent

Numerous studies have failed to demonstrate bacterial, viral or fungal infections as causative of IC (Hanash and Pool 1970; Hedelin et al. 1983). Hunner in 1915 originally proposed that IC was a result of chronic bacterial infection of the bladder (Hunner 1915).

The newest studies in this field investigated herpes simplex virus, but rendered a negative result (Fall 1985), and Epstein–Barr virus (Gillespie and Jones 1986).

In the latter study 118 of 150 patients with IC were found to have a marked elevation of certain anti-capsid antigen antibodies in the blood.

Antibiotics have been proposed as being able to induce IC, but it has not been convincingly proved. As IC commonly has a subacute or acute onset suggestive of urinary tract infection, it is reasonable to assume that most patients would sooner or later receive antibiotics. Nitrofurantoin and tetracycline have been proposed to be "surface active" drugs, which might interfere with the glycosaminoglycans layer lining the urothelium (Gillespie et al. 1985). It is well known that drugs may alter the rate of synthesis of mucus, the chemical and physical structure of mucus and its rate of secretion from epithelial cells and thereby affect the normal cytoprotection of the epithelium (Parke and Symmons 1977). However, the role of antibiotics in IC is yet to be clarified.

To further elucidate the role of an etiologic substance in the urine, our group has done several studies. The blood basophils are the counterpart of the tissue mast cells. The attraction of basophils to the inflammatory sites indicate that these cells play an important role in immune processes. We used urine from patients with IC and normal controls and incubated in vitro the urine with basophil leucocytes from the same patients and controls using the method measuring histamine liberation described by Stahl Skov (1983). The basophil leucocytes did not in any case liberate histamine indicating that no allergic type-I reaction is taking place due to a substance in the urine (Holm-Bentzen et al. unpublished results, 1986).

A study using epicutaneous reactions with urine was also performed (Clemmensen et al. 1988). The study showed that patients with IC had a high incidence of positive skin reactions to patch tests with urine compared to controls (Table 6.3). The positive reactions were primarily seen with the patients own urine, but also, although less frequently, with foreign urine. Immediate skin reactions were not seen. The morphology and histology of the positive patch tests suggested a toxic rather than an allergic reaction. These data support the assumption that urine contains a substance that elicits a probably toxic reaction in IC patients. This factor is found in increased amounts in urine from IC patients; furthermore these patients have a decreased threshold to the component, possibly due to a defective mucous layer of the bladder.

Table 6.3. Results after epicutaneous patch test reactions with urine in patients with interstitial cystitis and healthy controls

| | | Positive reactions | |
		Autologous urine[a]	Homologous urine
Patients	+ Stripping[b]	7	4
(n = 11)	− Stripping	4	0
Controls	+ Stripping	0	1
(n = 8)	− Stripping	0	0

[a] Autologous = own; homologous = foreign (patient and control urine respectively).
[b] Stripping, stratum corneum removed with adhesive tape.

The GAG layer and Urothelium in the Pathogenetic Process

The mucous surface coat lining the urothelium, with its content of glycosaminoglycans, is thought to play a role in the cytoprotection of the bladder (Parsons 1986) and acts as an important defense mechanism between the urothelial cells and bacteria and other harmful substances in the urine (Hanno et al. 1978). There are seven major classes of glycosaminoglycans (GAGs), earlier called acid mucopolysaccharides (Lamberg and Stoolmiller 1974; Hjelm Poulsen 1986): chondroitin 4- and 6-sulfate, dermatan sulfate, keratan sulfate, heparan sulfate, hyaluronic acid and heparin. GAGs in tissue are not free (except for hyaluronic acid) but always incorporated in proteoglycans together with a core protein. Proteoglycans are enormous molecules with a central hyaluronic acid string and approximately 40 proteoglycan manomers (molecular weight 10^9). One proteoglycan manomer consists of a core protein and different GAGs radiating outward (Höök et al. 1984; Comper and Laurent 1978). GAGs are distributed in the matrix of connective tissue all over the body, but the presence of GAGs on cell surfaces have now been demonstrated in several systems (Höök et al. 1984). GAGs are extremely hydrophilic because of their negatively charged compounds, and are therefore capable of forming a barrier between the surface and the environment (Gregor 1973).

Parsons was the first who drew attention to the relationship between IC and the GAG layer. It was hypothesized that patients with IC had a missing GAG layer, which was also the rationale for treating these patients with synthetic GAG (Parsons et al. 1982). These concepts have now been modified by recent studies (Holm-Bentzen et al. 1986).

Ultrastructural studies have failed to demonstrate morphological differences in the urothelium between IC patients and controls. (Collan et al. 1976). The most recent study using ruthenium red (Dixon et al. 1986) showed variations in the thickness of the GAG layer in different patients, but these differences were related to the surface topography of the luminal cell and there were no differences in variation between the IC patients and the normal controls (stress incontinent females) concerning the GAG layer. This morphologic study also showed that penetration of ruthenium red between surface urothelium cells down to the basement membrane occurred in a similar proportion of samples from both IC patients and controls, indicating this as a normal phenomenon. In an earlier Danish study (Eldrup et al. 1983), with colloidal lanthanum, differences in the permeability of the urothelium were demonstrated between IC patients and controls due to possible defective tight junctions. Lepinard also proposed that loss of the water-tight nature of the normal urothelium could be responsible for IC (Lepinard et al. 1984).

It still remains an open question as to how a normal urothelium is, and no data exist concerning the permeability of the basement membrane. Does the basement membrane act as a filter for possible harmful substances in the urine? Further studies are needed to clarify these questions.

It is now established that no morphologic changes are seen in the GAG layer in IC patients, but the GAG layer might still be quantitatively or qualitatively abnormal. If quantitative changes in the GAG layer are involved in the

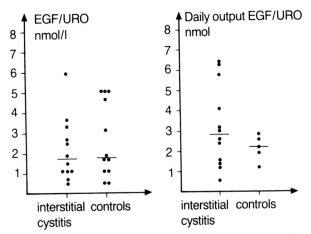

Fig. 6.2. The substance concentration and the daily output of EGF (epidermal growth factor) in urine from 12 patients with interstitial cystitis and 12 normal, age-matched controls.

pathogenesis of IC it is logical to hypothesize that the urothelial cells are producing smaller amounts of GAGs. EGF (epidermal growth factor or urogastrone) is a growth promoting hormone which plays a role in cytoprotection and the production of GAGs in the gastrointestinal tract (Olsen et al. 1984). We investigated the urinary excretion of EGF in IC patients but found no changes in the urinary excretion when compared to normal, age-matched controls (Holm-Bentzen et al. 1987b) (Fig. 6.2).

New quantitative studies in these patients deserve mentioning. Decreased urinary excretion of GAGs measured by the uronate content in patients with IC (3–36 nmol/ml uronate/ml urine) compared with controls (62–69 nmol/ml) has been shown (Hurst et al. 1985). Recently the same authors again proposed some interesting theories based on quantitative GAG studies (Hurst et al. 1986). They presented quantitative differences between urethral and bladder urine in IC patients and hypothesized that exogenous GAGs from the kidney might "patch" damaged areas on the bladder urothelium.

Qualitative studies on the GAG layer with lectin probes have shown that carbohydrate terminals of the bladder surface GAGs are unchanged in patients with IC, but that the bio-chemical compositions of the different GAGs are altered (more galactose and fucose in IC patients) (Sant et al. 1986).

In a preliminary study we investigated the qualitative differences in the mucous surface coat of the bladder between IC patients and controls (Holm-Bentzen et al. 1986). By a new cytoscopic scraping method the mucous surface coat including the GAGs were collected in a buffer and analysed by electrophoresis in a monodimension run, using the methods described in the literature (Moller et al. 1985; Cappelletti et al. 1979). We found that IC patients had a higher percentage of hyaluronic acid and dermatan sulfate in the mucous surface coat than controls (prostatic hypertrophy) (Fig. 6.3). The patients had a lack of heparan sulfate which is known to be the major GAG on cell surfaces (Comper and Laurent 1978).

All these studies seem to indicate that certain abnormalities do exist in the composition of the GAGs in the mucous surface coat in patients with IC and it is

Painful bladder   **Controls**

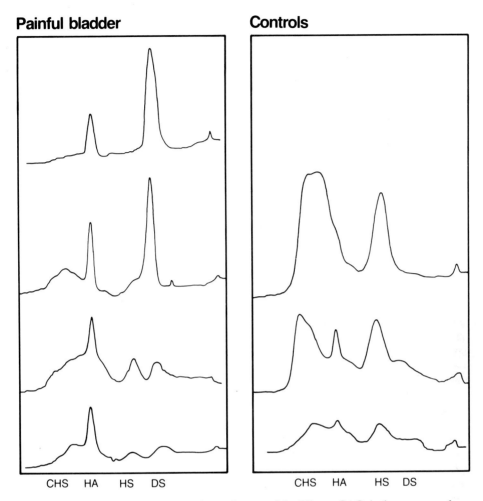

Fig. 6.3. The densitometric scans of the electrophoreses of the different GAGs in the mucous surface coat of the human urinary bladder in 4 patients with interstitial cystitis and 3 patients with prostatic hypertrophy (controls). CHS, chondroitin 4–6-sulfate; HA, hyaluronic acid; HS, heparan sulfate; DS, dermatan sulfate.

logical to conclude that an impaired cytoprotection plays a role in the pathogenesis of IC.

The Inflammatory Processes in the Bladder Wall

The exact nature of the inflammatory changes found in the bladder wall in IC patients still remains unclear. Pathoanatomically, there is a chronic inflammatory response with mononuclear cells and a varying degree of collagen deposits (fibrosis). The collagen is distributed in a characteristic fashion, namely with collagen inside the muscle fascicles (Larsen et al. 1982; Holm-Bentzen and Lose 1987). This is in contrast to the pattern of collagen infiltration in, for example, prostatic hypertrophy, where the collagen is distributed between the muscle fascicles (Gosling and Dixon 1980). Furthermore in IC, there is an infiltration of mast cells in the detrusor muscle. The degree of fibrosis is varying, but it is well known that some patients end up with a small, shrunken fibrotic bladder. The lamina propria in IC patients is edematous with mononuclear cell infiltrations and dilated vessels and some fibrosis. An elevated number of mast cells seem to be present here at least in some stages of the disease as mentioned earlier in this chapter.

We still do not know what initiates this chronic inflammatory response. Is it a reaction to a toxic agent, an allergen or is the process autoimmunological? Since the mast cells are so often in evidence, it is reasonable to believe that they play a role, and by an unknown mechanism are attracted from the blood to bladder tissue. Degranulation of the mast cells is induced and the different mediators are released: histamine, prostaglandins, chemotactic factors, leukotrienes, heparin, etc.

Recently many studies have been done trying to monitor the inflammatory response by measuring the released mediators or their derivatives. When eosinophilic chemotactic factor is released by the degranulating mast cells, eosinophils are mobilized to the inflammatory site, where they modify the inflammatory response through deposition of granule products including eosinophil cationic protein (ECP) and/or phagocytosis of mast cell granules (Venge et al. 1980). An increased number of eosinophils in bladder biopsies from patients with IC is found together with an increased concentration of ECP in urine (Lose 1985, Lose et al. 1987), compared with other patients with painful bladder disease (Table 6.4). ECP might be responsible for the maintenance of the inflammatory process and the tissue destruction in IC. ECP in urine was measured by a newly developed enzyme-immunoassay (Frandsen and Lose 1986).

An elevated urinary excretion of a metabolite of histamine, 1,4 methylimidazole acetic acid (1,4-MIAA), has also been demonstrated in IC patients (Holm-Bentzen et al. 1987a), (Fig. 6.4). 1,4-MIAA was measured by reversed phase ion-pair high performance liquid chromatography (Søndergaard 1982). An elevated concentration of histamine in bladder biopsies in IC patients was also demonstrated (Kastrup et al. 1983; Lynes et al. 1986). Another

Table 6.4. The number of mast cells in the detrusor, percentage of biopsies with eosinophilic infiltration, the peripheral eosinophil count and ECP concentration in urine in 15 patients with interstitial cystitis and 15 patients with other types of painful bladder diseases

	Interstitial cystitis	Other types of painful bladder disease
Mast cells/mm^2 in the detrusor (mean)	49	5
Percentage of biopsies with eosinophil infiltration	43%	4%
Eosinophils (10^7/1) (mean) (normal range <35)	10.2	11.5
ECP (eosinophil cationic protein) (U/1) (mean) (normal range 1–36 U/1)	140	14

1,4-MIAA, mg/24 h

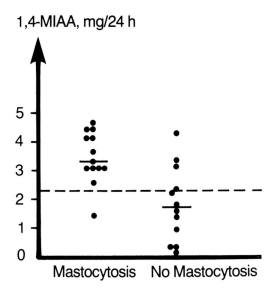

Mastocytosis   No Mastocytosis

Fig. 6.4. Urinary excretion of 1,4-methylimidazole acetic acid (1,4-MIAA) in 13 patients with interstitial cystitis and 12 patients with other types of painful bladder disease. (Median values are shown. Dashed line indicates upper limit normal range.)

mediator from mast cell degranulation, prostaglandin E_2, has also been found in elevated urinary concentrations in IC patients (Lynes et al. 1986).

Autoimmune reactions might explain many facets of interstitial cystitis and have been proposed as initiating the inflammatory response (Oravisto 1980). The pathological findings, the chronic but relapsing course of the disease and certain immunological studies would seem to indicate this. On the contrary, however, the way these patients respond to immunosuppression and anti-inflammatory drugs argues against it (Messing 1986). Also the recurrence of IC in colocystoplasties (McGuire et al. 1973) and the disappearance of symptoms after urinary diversion without cystectomy (Linder and Smith 1958), argues against the autoimmune theory. A high incidence of antinuclear antibodies in patients with IC has been reported, but the titers were low, less than 1:10 in half of the patients (Oravisto 1980; Oravisto et al. 1970). Oravisto also reported a high incidence of other hypersensitivity disorders in these patients. Others have identified circulating bladder antibodies in serum (Silk 1970; Gordon et al. 1973). Our group was unable to confirm these results in our IC patients (Hald and Holm-Bentzen 1986) but another Finnish study has given no support to the concept of an organospecific autoimmune disease (Jokinen et al. 1972b).

Mattila studied vascular immunopathology in 47 IC patients and found 33 with immune deposits in the bladder vascular wall (Mattila 1982). Severe endothelial damage compatible with immunologically induced changes was found in 14 out of 20 patients with IC in an electronmicroscopic study (Mattila et al. 1983a). Further studies by the Finnish group also suggest activation of complement to be involved (Mattila and Linder 1984; Mattila et al. 1983b). The association of IC with connective tissue diseases, especially lupus erythematosus, has also been speculative (Oravisto et al. 1970; Jokinen et al. 1972a; Weisman et al. 1981). In many ways IC resembles a local manifestation of lupus but there is no evidence for a systemic connective tissue disease.

In conclusion it must be stated that the exact nature of the inflammatory processes in the bladder wall has not been completely elicited. The degranulation of mast cells and the activation of eosinophils constitute a typical sequence of events in an IgE mediated Type-I hypersensitivity reaction, but still IC remains to be classified as an allergic disease. However, other stimuli may lead to mast cell degranulation (Tai and Spry 1981; Belsan and Bass 1977) and a Type-III and Type IV hypersensitivity reaction seem more likely to be responsible for the processes seen in the bladder wall in IC.

Neurogenic and Psychiatric Aspects of Etiology and Pathogenesis

There is sparse literature concerning the nerves in the bladder in patients with IC. The nerves have never been systematically investigated which is rather surprising since these patients' major symptom is bladder pain. In a normal urinary bladder the sensory nerve endings are free and unspecialized and distributed in the mucosa, submucosa and in the connective tissue between the detrusor muscle bundles (Bradley 1986). Some authors describe fibrosis around the nerve fibres as characteristic of the disease (Smith and Dehner 1972) and others describe perineural cell infiltration with inflammatory cells as an outstanding feature (Fall et al. 1985). Fall even describes relief of symptoms after resection of the affected nerves (Fall 1985). Our group observed the same perineural cell infiltration, but especially in the detrusor myopathy group of painful bladder patients (Holm-Bentzen et al. 1985).

Recently, some presumptive sensory nerves in the lamina propria adjacent to the urothelium in the human urinary bladder have been described (Dixon et al. 1984). These nerves may represent peripheral terminals of bladder sensory nerves and were morphologically clearly different from the nerve terminals in the muscle coat. There were no differences in number and morphology of these nerves in controls and patients with autonomic disorders (Shy-Drager syndrome, diabetic neuropathy, etc.) These nerves have not been studied in IC patients, and it is not known whether these nerves are proprioceptive (relaying information on tension and contraction) or exteroceptive (relaying information on pain, touch and temperature) (ICS definitions 1975, 1976).

The significance of neuropeptides in the function of the lower urinary tract is still not exactly evaluated (Mundy 1984). Substance P is found in subepithelial nerves in the human urinary bladder and vasoactive intestinal polypeptide (VIP) is suggested as an inhibitory neurotransmitter in the detrusor (Klarskov et al. 1987). In a preliminary study (Holm-Bentzen et al. 1987d) the concentration of VIP in bladder biopsies from painful bladder patients, with and without an elevated mast cell count, and controls was investigated, but no differences in the mean values of the VIP concentration were found (Fig. 6.5). VIP was measured by a radioimmunoassay (Fahrenkrug 1979). All mean values were around 10 pmol/g.

It has been quite common, even amongst urologists, to speculate that

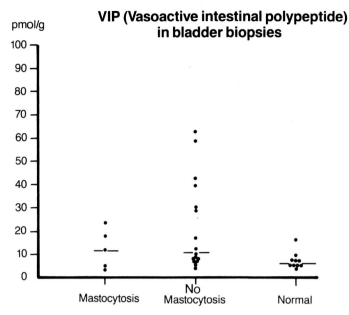

VIP (Vasoactive intestinal polypeptide) in bladder biopsies

Fig. 6.5. The concentration of VIP (pmol/g) in bladder biopsies in 5 patients with interstitial cystitis, 16 patients with other painful bladder diseases and 16 normals (stress incontinent females). (Mean values are shown.)

psychiatric abnormalities play a role in interstitial cystitis (Hand 1949). Some of these patients have been treated with success by means of bladder training (Blaivas and Blaivas 1986). We performed a study of 33 patients with IC, where a psychiatric interview and a Minnesota Multiphasic Personality Inventory (MMPI) were employed (unpublished results). The study showed that these patients exhibit a wide spectrum of psychiatric abnormalities (only 25% normal) and differ from the normal population in this respect. Only a few severe psychiatric abnormalities were found (Table 6.5). These findings were in agreement with studies of patients with chronic organic pain (Woodforde and Mersky 1972) and patients with other chronic bladder complaints (Macaulay et al. 1985). We therefore concluded that the psychiatric abnormalities in painful

Table 6.5. Psychiatric and psychological evaluation of 11 patients with interstitial cystitis and 22 patients with other painful bladder diseases

Diagnosis	Normal		Psychiatric vulnerable		Neurotic		Borderline		Psychotic/ psychopathic	
	Psych	MMPI	Psych	MMPI	Psych	MMPI	Psych	MMPI	Psych	MMPI
Interstitial cystitis	5	3	3	5	3	2	0	1	0	0
	45%	27%	27%	45%	27%	18%	0	9%	0	0
Other painful bladder diseases	10	5	6	11	6	2	0	4	0	0
	45%	23%	27%	50%	27%	9%	0	18%	0	0

Number of patients and percentages are shown. Psych, psychiatric interview; MMPI, Minnesota Multiphasic Personality Inventory.

bladder patients are more likely to be caused by the chronic pain and the voiding symptoms rather than being responsible for them. Furthermore, we did not find any difference between the patients with and without an elevated mast cell count in the detrusor and no correlation between the severity of the psychiatric abnormality and the severity of the bladder symptoms, the duration of the disease and the existence of a psychotrauma.

Conclusions

During the last few years IC has fortunately been the focus for a lot of very interesting research. There is a great demand from urologic patients that this research should continue. We still do not have the ideal treatment to offer these patients, however, since we still do not know the exact etiologic agents and pathogenetic mechanisms which lead to the disease. The other problems, as mentioned in the introduction, are the disagreement among physicians and urologists on how to define and diagnose the disease, or, more likely, the syndrome. In the future it is absolutely necessary for collaborative studies to clarify further this interesting, but for the patient very disabling disease.

References

Aldenborg F, Fall M, Enerbäck L (1985) Proliferation and transepithelial migration of mucosal mast cells in interstitial cystitis. Immunology 58:411–416

Belsan PB, Bass DA (1977) The eosinophil. Major problems in internal medicine. Saunders, Philadelphia, p 58

Blaivas S, Blaivas JG (1986) Successful treatment of sensory urgency and interstitial cystitis with behaviour modification. J Urol 135:189(A)

Borque JP (1951) Surgical management of the painful bladder. J Urol 65:25–30

Bradley WE (1986) Physiology of the urinary bladder. In: Walsh A et al. (eds) Cambell's urology, 4th edn, vol 1. Saunders, Philadelphia, p 129

Cappelletti R, Del Rosso M, Chiarugi VP (1979) A new electrophoretic method for the complete separation of all known animal glycosaminoglycans in a monodimensional run. Anal Biochem 99:311–315

Clemmensen O, Lose G, Holm-Bentzen M, Colstrup H (1988) Skin reactions to urine in patients with interstitial cystitis. Urology 32:17–20

Collan Y, Alfthan O, Kivilaakso E, Oravisto KJ (1976) Electron microscopic and histological findings in urinary bladder epithelium in interstitial cystitis. Eur Urol 2:242–247

Comper WD, Laurent TC (1978) Physiological function of connective tissue polysaccharides. Physiol Rev 58:255–316

Deane AM, Parkinson MC, Cameron KM, Hindmarsh JR (1983) Mast cells in female sensory bladder disorders. Proceedings of the International Continence Society, annual meeting, Aachen, p 51

Dixon JS, Gilpin SA, Gilpin CJ, Gosling JA (1984) Presumptive sensory nerves in the human urinary bladder. Proceedings of the International Continence Society, annual meeting, Innsbruck, p 272

Dixon JS, Holm-Bentzen M, Gilpin CJ et al. (1986) Electron microscopic investigation of the bladder urothelium and glycocalyx in patients with interstitial cystitis. J Urol 135:621–625

Eldrup J, Thorup J, Nielsen SL, Hald T, Hainau B (1983) Permeability and ultrastructure of human bladder epithelium. Br J Urol 55:488–492

Fahrenkrug J (1979) Vasoactive intestinal polypeptide: measurement, distribution and putative neurotransmitter function. Digestion 19:149–155

Fall M (1985) Conservative management of chronic interstitial cystitis: transcutaneous electrical nerve stimulation and transurethral resection. J Urol 133:774–778

Fall M, Johansson SL, Vahlne A (1985) A clinico-pathological and virological study of interstitial cystitis. J Urol 133:771–775

Feltis JT, Perez-Marrero R and Emerson LE (1985) Urinary bladder mast cell infiltrates in suspected cases of interstitial cystitis. J Urol 133:143A

Frandsen B, Lose G (1986) Determination of eosinophil cationic protein in urine by an enzyme immunoassay. Scand J Clin Lab Invest 46:629–632

Gillespie LM, Jones JF (1986) Epstein–Barr virus infection and interstitial cystitis: the rosetta stone of inflammatory disease? J Urol 135:271A

Gillespie LM, Said J, Cain D, Van der Veld R (1985) Antibiotic-induced interstitial cystitis: a model for cell membrane instability. Proceedings of the International Continence Society, annual meeting, London, p 254

Gordon HL, Rossen RD, Hersh EM and Yium JJ (1973) Immunologic aspects of interstitial cystitis. J Urol 109:228–233

Gosling JA, Dixon JS (1980) Structure of trabeculated detrusor smooth muscle in cases of prostatic hypertrophy. Urol Int 35:351–356

Gregor HP (1973) Anticoagulant activity of sulfonate polymers and copolymers. In: Gregor HP (ed) Polymer science and technology, vol 5. Plenum Press, New York, p 51

Hald T, Holm-Bentzen M (1986) Clinical symptom complex. In: George NJR, Gosling JA (eds) Sensory disorders of the bladder and urethra. Springer, Berlin Heidelberg New York, p 49

Hanash KA, Pool TL (1970) Interstitial and hemorrhagic cystitis: viral, bacterial and fungal studies. J Urol 104:705–706

Hand JR (1949) Interstitial cystitis: Report of 223 cases (204 women and 19 men). J Urol 61:291–310

Hanno PM, Fritz R, Wein AJ, Mulholland SG (1978) Heparin as antibacterial agent in rabbit bladder. Urology 12:411–415

Hedelin HH, Mårdh P-A, Brorson JE, Fall M, Moller B, Pettersson KGS (1983) Mycoplasma hominis and interstitial cystitis. Sex Transm Dis 10:327–330

Hellstrom HR, Davis BK, Shonnard JW (1979) Eosinophilic cystitis. A study of 16 cases. Am J Clin Pathol 72:777–785

Hjelm Poulsen J (1986) Urine and tissue glycosaminoglycans and their interrelations. Dan Med Bull 33:75–96

Holm-Bentzen M (1985) Painful bladder: classification of the disease. Scand J Urol Nephrol [Suppl] 94:10

Holm-Bentzen M, Lose G (1987) Pathology and pathogenesis of interstitial cystitis. Urology [Suppl] 29(4):8–13

Holm-Bentzen M, Larsen S, Hainau B, Hald T (1985) Non-obstructive detrusor myopathy in a group of patients with chronic abacterial cystitis. Scand J Urol Nephrol 19:21–26

Holm-Bentzen M, Ammitzbøll T, Hald T (1986) Glycosaminoglycans on the surface of the human urothelium: a preliminary report. Neurourol Urodyn 5:519–523

Holm-Bentzen M, Søndergaard I, Hald T (1987a) Urinary excretion of a metabolite of histamine (1,4-methyl-imidazole-acetic-acid) in painful bladder disease. Br J Urol 59:230–233

Holm-Bentzen M, Lose G, Jørgensen L, Sørensen K and Nexø E (1987b) Chronic cystitis: Excretion of epidermal growth factor (EGF)/urogastrone (URO). Urol Res 15:203–205

Holm-Bentzen M, Jacobsen F, Nerstrøm B et al. (1987c) Painful bladder disease: clinical and pathoanatomical differences in 115 patients. J Urol 137:500–502

Holm-Bentzen M, Jacobsen F, Nerstrøm B et al. (1987d) A prospective double-blind, clinically controlled, multicenter trial of Elmiron (sulpho-pentosan sodium) in the treatment of interstitial cystitis and related painful bladder diseases. J Urol 137:503–507

Holm-Bentzen M, Christensen JK, Lieth L and Hald T (1989) Psychiatric and psychological evaluation of patients with painful bladder. Neurourol Urodyn (in press)

Höök M, Kjellèn L, Johansson S, Robinson J (1984) Cell-surface glycosaminoglycans. Ann Rev Biochem 53:847–869

Hunner GL (1915) A rare type of bladder ulcer in women: report of cases. Boston Med Surg J 172:660–664

Hurst RE, Roy JB, Bynum RL, Parry WL (1985) Abnormal glycosaminoglycans excretion in patients with chronic interstitial cystitis. J Urol 133:144A

Hurst RE, Parsons CL, Roy JB (1986) The mechanisms for low glycosaminoglycans excretion in interstitial cystitis and mechanisms for protection of bladder from urine. J Urol 135:189A

Jokinen EJ, Lasssus A, Salo OP, Alfstan O (1972a) Discoid lupus erythematosus and interstitial cystitis. Ann Clin Res 4:23–25

Jokinen EJ, Alfthan OS, Oravisto KJ (1972b) Antitissue antibodies in interstitial cystitis. Clin Exp Immunol 11:333–339

Kastrup J, Hald T, Larsen S, Nielsen VG (1983) Histamine content and mast cell count of detrusor muscle in patients with interstitial cystitis and other types of chronic cystitis. Br J Urol 55:495–500

Klarskov P, Holm-Bentzen M, Nørgaard T, Ottosen B, Walther S, Hald T (1987) Vasoactive intestinal polypeptide concentration in human bladder-neck smooth muscle and its influence on urodynamic parameters. Br J Urol 60:113–118

Lamberg SI, Stoolmiller AC (1974) Glycosaminoglycans. A biochemical and clinical review. J Invest Dermatol 63:433–449

Larsen S, Thompson SA, Hald T et al. (1982) Mast cells in interstitial cystitis. Br J Urol 54:283–286

Lepinard V, Saint-Andre JP, Rogon LM (1984) La cystite interstitielle. J Urol (Paris) 90:455–465

Linder CH, Smith RD (1958) Hunner's ulcer. Br J Urol 30:338–342

Lose G (1985) Urine eosinophilic cationic proteins and complement in interstitial cystitis. Scand J Urol Nephrol [Suppl] 94:9–13

Lose G, Frandsen B, Holm-Bentzen M, Larsen S, Jacobsen F (1987) Urine eosinophilic cationic protein in painful bladder disease. Br J Urol 60:39–42

Lynes WL, Shortliffe LD, Flynn SA, Zipser R, Roberts J (1986) Mast cell involvement in interstitial cystitis. J Urol 135:272A

Macaulay AJ, Holmes D, Stanton SL, Stern RS (1985) A clinic survey of the mental state of 211 women attending a urodynamic unit. Proceedings of the International Continence Society, annual meeting, London, p 180

Mattila J (1982) Vascular immunopathology in interstitial cystitis. Clin Immun Immunopathol 23:648–652

Mattila J, Linder E (1984) Immunoglobin deposits in the bladder epithelium and vessels in interstitial cystitis: possible relationship to circulating anti-intermediate filament autoantibodies. Clin Immunol Immunopathol 3:81–89

Mattila J, Pitkanen R, Vaalasti T (1983a) Fine-structural evidence for vascular injury in patients with interstitial cystitis. Vircshows Arch 398:347–355

Mattila J, Harmoinen A, Hällström O (1983b) Serum immunoglobulin and complement alterations in interstitial cystitis. Eur Urol 9:350–353

McGuire ES, Lytton B, Carnog SL (1973) Interstitial cystitis following colocystoplasty. Urology 2:28–29

Messing EM (1986) Interstitial cystitis and related syndromes. In: Walsh A et al. (eds) Cambell's urology, 4th edn., vol 1. Saunders, Philadelphia, p 1070

Møller R, Serup J, Ammitzbøll T (1985) Glycosaminoglycans in localized scleroderma (Morphoea). Connect Tissue Res 13:227–230

Mundy AR (1984) Neuropeptides in lower urinary tract function. World J Urol 2:211–216

Olsen PS, Poulsen SS, Kirkegaard P, Nexø E (1984) Role of submandibular saliva and epidermal growth factor in gastric cytoprotection. Gastroenterology 87:103–108

Oravisto KJ (1980) Interstitial cystitis as an autoimmune disease. A review. Eur Urol 6:10–13

Oravisto KJ, Alfthan OS, Jokinen EJ (1970) Interstitial cystitis, clinical and immunological findings. Scand J Urol Nephrol 4:37–42

Parke DV, Symmons AM (1977) The biochemical pharmacology of mucus. Adv Exp Med Bio 89:423–441

Parsons CL (1986) Bladder surface glycosaminoglycans: efficient mechanism of environmental adaption. Urology [Suppl] 27:9–14

Parsons CL, Schmidt JD, Pollen JJ (1983) Successful treatment of interstitial cystitis with sodium pentosan polysulfate. J Urol 130:51–54

Sant GR, Ucci AA, Alroy J (1986) Bladder surface glycosaminoglycans (GAGs) in interstitial cystitis. J Urol 135:175A

Silk MR (1970) Bladder antibodies in interstitial cystitis. J Urol 103:307–309

Smith B, Dehner LP (1972) Chronic ulcerating interstitial cystitis. A study of 28 cases. Arch Pathol 93:76–81

Søndergaard I (1982) Quantitative determination of 1,4-methyl-imidazole-acetic-acid in urine by high performance liquid chromatography. Allergy 37:581–584

Stahl Skov P (1983) The allergic type-I reaction. In vitro studies on human basophile leucocytes and rat mast cells. Medical thesis, University of Copenhagen

Tai PC, Spry CSF (1981) The mechanisms which produce vacuolated and degranulated eosinophils. J Haematol 49:211–214

Venge P, Dahl R, Hällgren R, Olsson I (1980) Cationic proteins of human eosinophils and their role in the inflammatory reaction. In: Mahmoud AAF, Austen KF (eds) The eosinophils in health and disease. Grune and Stratton, New York

Wein A (1985) "Tell her to get a urine culture, take some of that medicine I prescribed a while ago and call me in a few days", Neurourol Urodynam 4:153–155 (editorial)

Weisman MH, McDanald EC, Wilson CB (1981) Studies of the pathogenesis of interstitial cystitis, obstructive uropathy, and intestinal malabsorption in a patient with systemic lupus erythematosus. Am J Med 70:875–878

Woodforde JM, Mersky H (1972) Personality traits of patients with chronic pain. J Psychosom Res 16:167–172

Editorial Comment

Etiologic Theories: Deficiency of the Bladder Lining

D. Staskin

The possibility that interstitial cystitis results from a defective barrier between the urine and the bladder epithelium allowing "normal" or toxic subsances to penetrate the bladder lining has been suggested but has not been substantiated.

Parsons and co-workers (1983) suggested that a deficiency of the glyco-saminoglycan (GAG) layer allows normally excluded (but not specified) agents within the urine to reach the deeper layers of the bladder. The symptomatic response of patients to sodium pentosanpolysulfate (SP-54), an oral heparin analog which is believed to supplement this lining, is used to support this hypothesis. No studies performed to date, however, demonstrate a deficiency of the GAG layer in these patients or a regeneration of the GAG layer in patients who respond to SP-54 therapy.

Dixon and co-workers (1986) presented the results of electron microscopic studies of the bladder urothelium and glycocalyx in 10 patients with well defined interstitial cystitis (pain, frequency every 1–3 hours and nocturia 3–12, submucosal hemorrhage on hydrodistension, and greater than 28 mast cells/ mm^2) but demonstrated no differences in the morphologic appearance of the glycocalyx or urothelial cells in patients with interstitial cystitis compared with controls. These authors did not, however, rule out a qualitative change in the GAG layer which may exist in interstitial cystitis but may have been imperceptible by the staining technique which was utilized.

Fowler and co-workers (1988) have demonstrated evidence for a defective mucosal barrier. Utilizing immunohistochemical techniques, they assayed for intraurothelial Tamm–Horsfall protein (THP). Ten of 14 patients with a clinical diagnosis of interstitial cystitis as opposed to 1 of 10 patients without the diagnosis of interstitial cystitis, demonstrated the presence of THP in the superficial cell layer. Intracellular THP could not be ruled out and no THP was seen adjacent to the luminal surface. Of interest, however, is that no THP was noted in the intermediate or basal cell layers of the urothelium, or in the submucosal or detrusor. The mean mast cell densities in the biopsies associated with THP were greater than in biopsies without THP but the differences were not statistically significant.

References

Dixon JS, Holm-Bentzen M, Gilpin CJ et al. (1986) Electron microscopic investigation of the bladder urothelium and glycocalyx in patients with interstitial cystitis. J Urol 135:621–624
Fowler JE, Lynes WL, Lau JLT, Ghosn L, Mounzer A (1988) Interstitial cystitis is associated with intraurothelial Tamm–Horsfall protein. J Urol 140:1385–1389
Parsons CL, Schmidt JD, Pollen JY (1983) Successful treatment of interstitial cystitis with sodium pentosanpolysulfate. J Urol 130:51–53

Section 3

Diagnosis

Chapter 7

Light Microscopic Findings in Bladders of Patients with Interstitial Cystitis

S.L. Johansson

In recent years it has been demonstrated that interstitial cystitis (IC) is more of a syndrome than a specific disease entity (Fall et al. 1987). Most urologists establish the diagnosis by a triad of clinical findings which include:

1. Characteristic irritative voiding symptoms including urgency and pain
2. The absence of objective evidence of other diseases that could cause these symptoms (including sterile urine)
3. Atypical cystoscopic appearance which generally is demonstrated with the patient under anesthesia (Messing 1987)

In patients with these symptoms two different cystoscopic appearances have been identified. The first patient category includes patients with an ulcer disease, as initially described by Hunner (1918). The second patient category does not display any ulcerations of the bladder mucosa, only strawberry-like hemorrhages, referred to as glomerulations. Patients with these features, which were initially described by Messing and Stamey in 1978, were said to suffer from "early interstitial cystitis." Practically all subsequent studies of interstitial cystitis have failed to subclassify the patients according to the two different cystoscopic patterns. The histopathologic findings in patients with IC generally have been described as nonspecific (Smith and Dehner 1972: Messing and Stamey 1978). Furthermore, many urologists, especially in the USA, do not obtain transurethral resection biopsies but only forcep or cold cut biopsies, which markedly limit the material available for histopathological evaluation.

Systematic evaluation of 128 patients, 64 of which were classic ulcerative IC cases, 44 with "early" IC, and 20 controls was performed (Johansson and Fall 1989). Four patients with ulcer disease were men and 60 were women, mean age at biopsy was 64 years (range 26–84 years). Four of the nonulcer patients were males, the other 40 were females, the mean age being 39 years (range 24–66 years).

The 20 control patients were all women, mean age 49 years (range 29–66 years). The biopsies were obtained by transurethral resection and generally included half of the detrusor muscle. The strips measured 0.5–1.5 cm and were obtained after the second distension from areas with ulcers, glomerulations, and

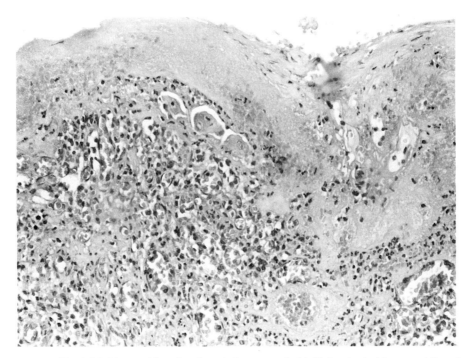

Fig. 7.1. Classic IC: Biopsy with wedge-shaped ulcer covered with fibrin mixed with neutrophils and erythrocytes. Note the granulation tissue present to the left of the ulcer. (H&E, original magnification ×33)

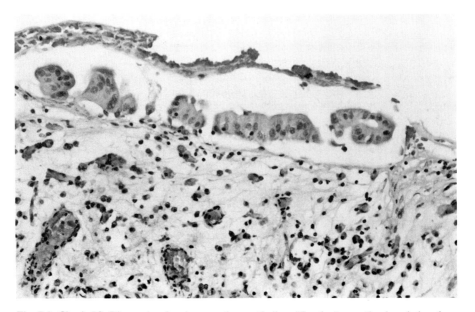

Fig. 7.2. Classic IC: Biopsy showing degenerative urothelium "floating" over the denuded surface. (H&E, original magnification ×66)

frequently also from cystoscopically normal mucosa. Nine patients with ulcer IC were subsequently subjected to total or subtotal cystectomy. The tissue was fixed either in 4% buffered formaldehyde or isosmotic mixture of 0.6% formaldehyde and 0.5% acetic acid (IFAA). Besides conventional staining with hematoxylin and eosin, sections were also stained with toluidine blue pH 0.5 for 30 min (IFAA embedded specimens). The formalin- fixed specimens were stained with toluidine blue for 5 days at pH 0.5 (Enerbäck, 1985). Blind evaluation of the specimens revealed very distinct and different histopathologic findings in the different groups. All patients with classic disease had ulcerated bladder mucosa. The ulcers frequently were wedge-shaped, usually covered by a mixture of fibrin, red blood cells and inflammatory cells (Fig. 7.1). The ulcers involved most of the lamina propria. The urothelium was either completely missing or seen "floating" above the bladder surface (Fig. 7.2). Interestingly enough, biopsies from areas of mucosa of normal appearance showed degenerative changes of the urothelium with ballooned cytoplasm, frequently with vacuolization. Of the patients with ulcer disease, 94% also exhibited granulation tissue which was composed of capillaries in a loose stroma with inflammatory cells and/or erythrocytes (see Fig. 7.1). The appearance of the granulation tissue was indistinguishable from granulation tissue elsewhere in the body. It is possible that distension during the normal filling phase results in rupture of the urothelium and exposure of the lamina propria to urine with formation of granulation tissue. Another striking finding was the presence of an intense mononuclear filtrate with over 90% of the patients having a dense 2+ to 3+ inflammatory mononuclear cell infiltrate (Fig. 7.3). Snap frozen specimens from 24 patients with classic IC were stained with a panel of monoclonal T- and

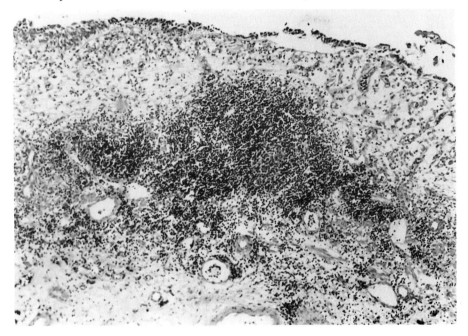

Fig. 7.3. Classic IC: Biopsy showing focal denuded mucosa and dense mononuclear inflammatory infiltrate. (H&E, original magnification ×33)

B-cell markers and compared with samples from nine patients with nonulcer IC and ten control patients. Control patients exhibited a minimal number of lymphoid cells, predominantly T-helper cells, rare B and plasma cells, and a normal T-helper to suppressor ratio. The nonulcer patients had small infiltrates of predominantly T-cells with focal aggregates, lacked B-cell nodules and had normal or increased T-helper to suppressor ratio. The lymphoid infiltrates of the classic patients were predominantly T-cells but also contained B-cell germinal centers and B- and T-cell nodules, focal clusters of plasma cells, and displayed a normal or decreased T-helper to suppressor ratio. The "nonulcer" patients differed from the controls in that T-cells and aggregates (greater than three cells) could easily be found which were not present in control patients. All of the ulcer patients had B-cell nodules which were not evident in the nonulcer group (Harrington et al. 1990).

Perineural and perivascular lymphocytic infiltrates have been identified in 80%–100% of the classic IC patients (Hand 1949; Smith and Dehner 1972; Fall et al. 1985; Johansson and Fall 1990). These infiltrates were markedly focal and varied in severity (Fig. 7.4). Perineural inflammatory infiltrates were almost never identified in forceps and/or cold cup biopsies because of the more superficial nature and relatively limited size of these biopsies.

Involvement of the mast cell system in patients with IC has been reported previously (Bohne et al. 1962). In our studies, mast cells counts demonstrated that only patients with classic IC had significantly increased numbers. Thus, in this patient category there were 164 mast cells per square millimeter in the lamina propria compared with 93 in the nonulcer IC group and 88 in the control groups ($P < 0.01$) (Johansson and Fall 1990). The mast cells in the detrusor

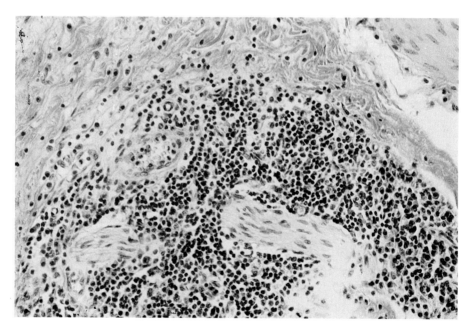

Fig. 7.4. Classic IC: Biopsy with marked perineural inflammatory infiltrate. (H&E, original magnification ×96)

muscle in patients with classic IC were more than doubled compared with nonulcer, 99 versus 46. The control patients had 36 mast cells per square millimeter. The majority of the patients with classic IC also had intraurothelial mast cells. The same patient category has also been shown to have abundant mast cells in bladder washing (Aldenborg et al. 1986). In recent years, there have been a number of studies reporting increased mast cells in patients with IC (Collan et al. 1976; Larsen et al. 1982; Kastrup et al. 1983; Lynes et al. 1987). Larsen et al. (1982) suggested that a finding of 28 mast cells per square millimeter in the detrusor muscle was indicative of IC and this has been used as a criteria for diagnosis in some studies of patients with painful bladder (Holm-Bentzen et al. 1987). However, in our experience most control patients had figures above 28 mast cells per square millimeter. The differences are probably best explained by the fact that we have used IFAA fixation, which prevents aldehyde blocking (Enerbäck 1966) or 5-day toluidine blue staining on formalin-fixed tissue which breaks the dye blocking and allows visualization of mucosal mast cells (Enerbäck 1966, 1967). A distinct property of mucosal mast cells both in rodents and man is susceptibility to aldehyde fixatives such as formalin (Enerbäck 1987). Thus, studies using formalin-fixed tissue and conventional toluidine blue stain, naphthol ASD chloroacetate (Leder) or Giemsa stain have failed to visualize this phenotypic population of mast cells.

Significant fibrosis was seen in less than 15% of the patients, predominantly in the cystectomy patients with classic IC. IC has generally been said to be a pancystitis. However, in our material the inflammatory, ulcerative changes involved the urothelium and the lamina propria. In the deeper parts of the bladder wall only mast cells were increased in the muscle layers and occasional focal perineural infiltrates were present. Only in three patients was there a true pancystitis. The overall inflammatory pattern seen in the majority of patients with classic IC is strikingly similar to that seen in patients with ulcerative colitis, a similarity which has been pointed out already by Bohne et al. (1962).

The patients with nonulcer IC displayed remarkably few and discrete histopathological changes, especially when taking into account that these patients had as severe symptomatology as the ulcer patients. Careful evaluation of biopsy material revealed that almost all of these patients had mucosal ruptures (Fig. 7.5). It seems very likely that these lesions were real and not artifacts, since they did not appear in control patients who had undergone completely identical procedure and biopsy. The ruptures occurred during distension of the bladder with a pressure of 70 cm of water. Since there was no inflammatory response or granulation tissue present, the ruptures or mucosal tears may have been the result of a defect in the cohesion of the urothelial lining cells resulting in the development of the rupture at this pressure. It was not possible to identify mucosal ruptures in a few cases, but very probably this was related to sampling and/or histological sectioning as well as the relatively limited size of these lesions. Besides the rupture, the nonulcer patients also had suburothelial hemorrhages corresponding to glomerulations, which were seen in almost 91% of the patients (Fig. 7.6). Ruptures and suburothelial hemorrhages were frequently seen in close proximity to each other (Fig. 7.7). By definition, glomerulations should be present in all patients, but they are frequently very small and may escape histologic detection.

Clinically, the differential diagnoses in patients with IC include bacterial cystitis. However, these patients have a urine sediment with numerous

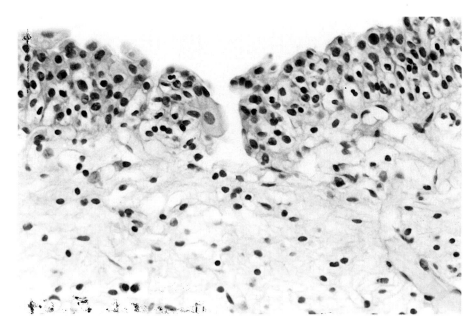

Fig. 7.5. Nonulcer IC: Biopsy displaying mucosal rupture. Note edema and absence of inflammatory response. H&E, original magnification ×96)

neutrophils, usually in association with abundant bacteria, whereas the sediment of patients with IC lacks these features. Patients with bacterial cystitis, for obvious reasons, should not be subjected to biopsy. Carcinoma in situ may sometimes be associated with symptoms similar to IC and endoscopically there

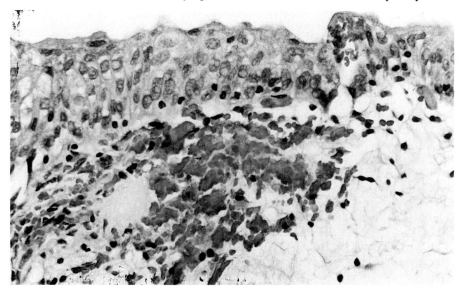

Fig. 7.6. Nonulcer IC: Biopsy with early rupture and suburothelial hemorrhage. (H&E, original magnification ×96)

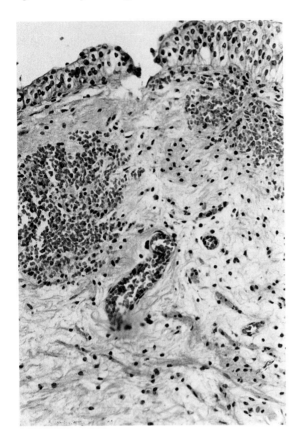

Fig. 7.7. Nonulcer IC: Biopsy with mucosal rupture and "glomerulations." (H&E, original magnification ×66)

may be similarities; however, this condition, has a quite different cytological and histological appearance. The main differential diagnosis that we have encountered is tuberculous cystitis, which can be associated with symptoms and histopathologic features very similar to classic IC. Granulomas may be sparse and it may be necessary to cut several levels to identify them, as well as to obtain cultures of the urine for mycobacteria.

Thus, in summary, the two different cytoscopic appearance of IC have characteristic light microscopic features. Patients with a classic (ulcer) IC display very characteristic features which includes mucosal ulceration with granulation tissue, hemorrhage, a marked mononuclear inflammatory infiltrate, increased mast cells in the lamina propria and the detrusor muscle, along with intraurothelial mast cells and perineural inflammatory infiltrates. The diagnosis of the ulcer disease is generally very easy on the light microscopic examination. In contrast, nonulcer patients display discrete morphologic changes which are dominated by mucosal ruptures and suburothelial hemorrhages, and these subtle lesions may be easily overlooked in a small biopsy. Therefore, these biopsies are generally identified as "mild to chronic inflammation and edema." Multiple sections and close scrutiny may help in the evaluation of these lesions.

Even though mast cells may be of the utmost importance in the pathogenesis of classic IC, special stains for these cells and techniques for counting them are not necessary in the routine diagnosis of IC.

References

Aldenborg F, Fall M, Enerbäck L (1986) Proliferation and transepithelial migration of mucosal mast cells in interstitial cystitis. Immunology 58:411–416

Bohne AW, Hodson JM, Roebuck JW, Reinhard RE (1962) An abnormal leukocyte response in interstitial cystitis. J Urol 88:387–391

Collan Y, Alfthan O, Kivilaakso E, Oravisto KJ (1976) Electron microscopic and histological findings on urinary bladder epithelium in interstitial cystitis. Eur Urol 2:242–247

Enerbäck L (1966) Mast cells in rat gastrointestinal mucosa. 1. Effect of fixation. Acta Pathol Microbiol Scand 66:298–302

Enerbäck L (1966) Mast cells in rat gastrointestinal mucosa. 2. Dye-binding and metachromatic properties. Acta Pathol Microbiol Scand 66:303–312

Enerbäck L (1985) Properties and function of mucosal mast cells. In: Gannelin CR, Schwartz JC (eds) Frontiers in histamine research. Pergamon, Oxford, pp 289ff

Enerbäck L (1987) Mucosal mast cells in the rat and man. Int Arch Allergy Appl Immunol 82:249–255

Fall M, Johansson SL, Vahlne A (1985) A clinopathologic and virologic study of interstitial cystitis. J Urol 133:771–773

Fall M, Johansson SL, Aldenborg F (1987) Chronic interstitial cystitis. A heterogenous syndrome. J Urol 137:35–38

Hand JR (1949) Interstitial cystitis: report of 233 cases. J Urol 61:291–310

Harrington DS, Fall M, Johansson SL (1990) Interstitial cystitis: bladder mucosa lymphocyte immunophenotyping and peripheral blood flow cytometry analysis. J Urol (in press)

Holm-Bentzen M, Jacobsen F, Nerstrom B et al. (1987) Painful bladder disease: clinical and pathoanatomical differences in 115 patients. J Urol 138:500–502

Hunner GL (1918) Elusive ulcer of the bladder. Am J Obstet 78:374–395

Johansson SL, Fall M (1990) Clinical features and spectrum of light microscopic changes in the bladders of patients with interstitial cystitis. J Urol (in press)

Kastrup J, Hald T, Larsen S, Nielsen VG (1983) Histamine content and mast cell count of detrusor muscle in patients with interstitial cystitis and other types of chronic cystitis. Br J Urol 55:495–500

Larsen S, Thompson SA, Hald T et al. (1982) Mast cells in interstitial cystitis. Br J Urol 54:283–286

Lynes WL, Flynn SD, Shortliffe LD et al. (1987) Mast cell involvement in interstitial cystitis. J Urol 138:746–752

Messing EM (1987) The diagnosis of interstitial cystitis. Urology 29:4–7

Messing EM, Stamey TA (1978) Interstitial cystitis: early diagnosis, pathology, and treatment. Urology 12:381–392

Smith B, Dehner LP (1972) Chronic ulcerating interstitial cystitis. A study of 28 cases. Arch Pathol 93:76–81

Chapter 8

Pathology of Interstitial Cystitis

J. Mattila

Histopathologically interstitial cystitis (IC) usually displays signs of nonspecific inflammation. The bladder epithelium is often injured, and was totally absent in 10 out of 47 IC patients (Mattila 1982). Similar findings are reported in other papers (Hand 1949; Franksson 1957; Oravisto et al. 1970: Smith and Dehner 1972; Jacobo et al. 1974; Skoluda et al. 1974). In 18 cases out of the 47 studied a chronic-type inflammation with lymphocytes and plasma cells could be seen. The cellular infiltrates were mostly located in the stromal tissue under the epithelium, and around the blood vessels. The vessel walls were often thickened. Hand (1949) also reported thickened vessel walls with narrowed lumen, and Franksson (1957) arteritis-like changes. Mast cells were more often seen in patients with IC than in control patients. An increased number of mast cells is also reported by others (Jacobo et al. 1974; Collan et al. 1976; De Juana and Everett 1977; Larsen et al. 1982). In nine cases inactive fibrosis or dilated vessels with thickened walls were observed. Twenty out of 47 biopsies were histologically normal.

Immunohistologically (Mattila 1982; Mattila and Linder 1984) more than 10% of IC patients had IgM deposits in the bladder epithelium. Immunoglobulins, mostly of IgM class, were found in the vessel walls of the bladder in 53% of IC patients, usually together with complement components C_{1q}, C_3 and C_4. Eight out of the 47 had only complement components and three patients only IgM deposits in the vascular walls. Deposits were focal, either encircling the entire vascular walls, or often segmental. IgM deposits in the vessel walls seemed to be associated partly with the endothelium and partly with the median cell structures and elastin elements.

Using electron microscopy we found severe endothelial injury in 14 out of 20 IC patients, and 10 patients showed smooth muscle injury in vessel walls. Additionally, clumps of elastic microfibrils of about 10 nm in diameter were seen in vessel walls. Electron-dense formations suggestive of immune deposits were occasionally seen in the subendothelial space. Medium-sized vessels containing elastic fibers and some layers of smooth muscle cells were, for the most part, injured (Mattila et al. 1983a).

A few papers include the results of electron microscopy of the bladder mucosa, particularly of the blood vessel walls. Skoluda et al. (1974) found lymphocyte and plasma cell infiltrates and fragmentation of plasma cells pointing to a mild immunologic process. The epithelium was often severely injured and the number of tonofilaments increased. Lymphocytes were seen in and beneath the epithelium. Narrowing of vessels due to swollen endothelial cells was seen. Collan et al. (1976) reported subepithelial capillaries with strongly thickened basement membranes together with large swollen epithelial cells with a decreased number of lateral processes in half of their 50 IC samples. Inflammatory changes were also seen in the mucosa. Boye et al. (1979) found multilayered endothelial basement membranes and noted that the sub-endothelial connective tissue compartment was regularly widened, containing amorphous material of variable electron density.

Under immunoelectron microscopy (IEM) we found in vivo bound IgM together with complement C_3 deposited in subendothelial spaces and in endothelial basement membranes, and associated with elastic fiber microfibrils (Helin et al. 1987).

The controversy as to the presence (Gordon et al. 1973; Lange 1975; Boye et al. 1979; Weissman et al. 1981) or absence (Skoluda et al. 1954; Jokinen et al. 1972b) or in vivo bound immune deposits in IC may be explained by the focal distribution of deposits seen in our study and, to some extent, by differences in methodology such as handling and fixation of tissue (Laurila et al. 1978).

In the case of circulating autoantibodies bladder specificity has not been studied (Gordon et al. 1973; Silk 1970) or established (Jokinen et al. 1972a).

We detected circulating autoantibodies to cytoskeletal intermediate filaments (IMFs) in IC patients (Mattila and Linder 1984). IMFs belong to the cytoskeleton of eukaryotic cell. Only IC patients had autoantibodies in high titer compared with controls. IMF-autoantibodies reacted in vitro with both bladder epithelium and vascular endothelium, in similar locations to those in which deposits were found in vivo. We do not know whether the anti-IMF-autoantibodies bind the bladder tissue in vivo and whether they are included in the deposits demonstrated by IEM. This seems possible, however, since antigenic similarities have been demonstrated between intracellular IMFs and extracellular microfibrils of developing elastic tissue (Linder et al. 1978a).

The role of anti-IMF-autoantibodies found in many diseases is still largely unknown. Some authors have stressed the association between autoantibodies and the development of pathologic states (Oldstone 1972; Linder et al. 1981; Dellagi et al. 1982; Dales et al. 1983). However, autoantibodies to IMFs also occur in normal human sera usually in low titers (Hintner 1983; Senegal et al. 1982; Linder and Lehto 1978b). This may be due to the fact that tissues are normally in a dynamic state of breakdown and synthesis. The amount of released tissue antigens is, however, too small to initiate a noticeable immune response (Allison and Denman 1976).

Our findings stress the immunologic aspects in the pathogenesis of interstitial cystitis. Cytoskeletal IMFs exposed in severe epithelial, endothelial and smooth muscle injuries and/or elastic microfibrils could act as antigens and initiate a tissue-damaging immune reaction. The vascular deposition of immunoglobulin and complement suggests that the vascular injury in IC is immunologically mediated (Cochrane and Koffler 1973; Williams 1981). The presence of C_3 together with early components of the classic pathway, C_{1q} and C_4 as well as the decreased serum levels of complement component C_4 (Mattila et al. 1983b) suggest classic complement pathway activation.

The autoantibodies directed to IMFs by the formation of immune complexes together with complement activation may contribute to tissue damage, and this would lead to the chronic self-perpetuating inflammation typical of this disease. A putative initial cytopathic factor, exposing intracytoplasmic structures, has to be postulated. The bladder epithelium, as well as the vascular endothelium, may be targets for microbial or toxic damage as a primary event and the liberated IMFs may subsequently give rise to autoantibody formation. Virus infections in particular have been regarded potential triggering mechanisms for autoimmunization, causing the chronic type of injury as a secondary event (Allison 1973: Glynn 1975). The relationship between viral infection (Toh et al. 1979; Linder et al. 1979; Bretherton and Toh 1981) and anti-IMF antibody responses is particularly interesting and only partially understood (Fujinami et al. 1983).

References

Allison AC (1973) Heberden Oration, 1972. Mechanisms of tolerance and autoimmunity. Ann Rheum Dis 32:282–293

Allison AC, Denman AM (1976) Self-tolerance and autoimmunity. Br Med Bull 32:124–129

Boye E, Morse M, Huttner I, Erlanger BF, McKinnon KJ, Classen J (1979) Immune-complex mediated interstitial cystitis as a major manifestation of systematic lupus erythematosus. Clin Immunol Immunopathol 13:67–76

Bretherton L, Toh BH (1981) IgM autoantibody to intermediate filaments in infectious mononucleosis. J Clin Lab Immuno 5:7–10

Cochrane CG, Koffler D (1973) Immune complex disease in experimental animals and man. Adv Immunol 16:185–264

Collan Y, Alfthan O, Kivilaakso E, Oravisto KJ (1976) Electron microscopic and histological findings on urinary bladder epithelium in interstitial cystitis. Eur Urol 2:242–247

Dales S, Fujinari RS, Oldstone MBA (1983) Infection with vaccinia favours the selection of hybridomas synthesizing autoantibodies against intermediate filaments, one of them cross-reacting with the virus hemagglutinin. J Immunol 1312:1546–1553

De Juana CP, Everett JC (1977) Interstitial cystitis. Urology 10:325–329

Dellagi K, Brouet JC, Perreau J, Paulin D (1982) Human monoclonal IgM with autoantibody activity against intermediate filaments. Proc Natl Acad Sci USA 79:446–450

Franksson C (1957) Interstitial cystitis: a clinical study of fifty-nine cases. Acta Chir Scand 113:51–62

Fujinami RS, Oldstone MBA, Wroblewska Z, Frankel ME, Koprowsky H (1983) Molecular mimicry in virus infection; crossreaction of measles virus phophorprotein or of herpes simplex virus protein with human intermediate filaments. Proc Natl Acad Sci USA 80:2346–2350

Glynn LE (1975) Experimental models and etiology of inflammatory rheumatic diseases. Scand J Rheumatol 5:55–62

Gordon HL, Rossen RD, Hersh EM, Yium JJ (1973) Immunologic aspects of interstitial cystitis. J Urol 109:228–233

Hand JR (1949) Interstitial cystitis. Report of 223 cases (204 women and 19 men). J Urol 61:291–310

Helin H, Mattila J, Rantala I (1984) In vivo binding of immunoglobulin and complement to elastic structures in urinary bladder vessel walls in interstitial cystitis: demonstration by immunoelectronmicroscopy. Clin Immunol Immunopathol 43:88–96

Hintner H, Steinert PM, Lawley TJ (1983) Human upper epidermal cytosplasmic antibodies are directed against keratin intermediate filaments. J Clin Invest 7:1344–1351

Jacobo E, Stamler FW, Culp DA (1974) Interstitial cystitis followed by total cystectomy. Urology 3:481–485

Jokinen EJ, Alfthan OS, Oravisto KJ (1972a) Antitissue antibodies in interstitial cystitis. Clin Exp Immunol 11:333–339

Jokinen EJ, Lassus A, Salo OP, Alfthan O (1972b) Discoid lupus erythematosus and interstitial cystitis. Ann Clin Res 4:23–25

Lange D (1975) Cystite interstitielle auto-immune. J Urol Nephrol 81:603–604

Larsen S, Thompsen SA, Hald T et al. (1982) Mast cells in interstitial cystitis. Br J Urol 54:283–286

Laurila P, Virtanen I, Vartiovaara J, Stenman S (1987) Fluorescent antibodies and lectins stain intracellular structures in fixed cell treated with nonionic detergent. J Histochem Cytochem 26:251–257

Linder E, Hormia M, Lehto V-P, Törnroth T (1981) Identification of cytoskeletal intermediate filaments in vascular endothelial cells as targets for autoantibodies in patient sera. Clin Immunol Immunopathol 21:217–227

Linder E, Kurki P. Anderson LC (1979) Autoantibody to "intermediate filaments" in infectious mononucleosis. Clin Immunol Immunopathol 14:411–417

Linder E, Lehto V-P, Kurki P, Stenman S, Virtanen I (1978a) Antigenic similarities between intracellular 10 nm filaments of fibroblasts and extracellular microfibrils of developing connective tissue. Prot Biol Fluids 26:621–627

Linder E, Lehto V-P (1978b) Antibodies against microfibrils of developing connective tissue in patients with inflammatory conditions. Scand J Immunol 7:239–244

Mattila J (1982) Vascular immunopathology in interstitial cystitis. Clin Immunol Immunopathol 23:648–655

Mattila J, Linder E (1984) Immunoglobulin deposits in bladder epithelium and vessels in interstitial cystitis: possible relationship to circulating anti-intermediate filament autoantibodies. Clin Immunol Immunopathol 323:81–89

Mattila J, Pitkänen R, Vaalasti T, Seppänen J (1983a) Fine-structural evidence for vascular injury in patients with interstitial cystitis. Virchows Arch 398:347–355

Mattila J, Harmoinen A, Hällström O (1983b) Serum immunoglobulin and complement alterations in interstitial cystitis. Eur Urol 9:350–352

Oldstone MBA (1972) Virus-induced autoimmune disease; viruses in the production and prevention of autoimmune disease. In: Day SB, Good RA (eds) Membranes and viruses in immunopathology. Academic Press, New York, pp 468–475

Oravisto KJ, Alfthan OS, Jokinen EJ (1970) Interstitial cystitis. Clinical and immunological findings. Scand J Urol Nephrol 4:37–42

Senegal JL, Rothfield NF, Oliver JM (1982) Immunoglobulin M autoantibody to vimentin intermediate filaments. J Clin Invest 69:716–721

Silk MR (1970) Bladder antibodies in interstitial cystitis. J Urol 103:307–309

Skoluda D, Wagner K, Lemmel EM (1974) Kritische Bemerkungen zur Immunopathogenese der interstitiellen Cystitis. Urologe (A) 13:15–23

Smith BH, Dehner LP (1972) Chronic ulcerating interstitial cystitis (Hunner's ulcer). Arch Pathol 93:76–81

Toh BH, Yildiz A, Sotelo J et al. (1979) Viral infections and IgM autoantibodies to cystoplasmic intermediate filaments. Clin Exp Immunol 37:76–82

Weissman MH, McDonald EC, Wilson CB (1981) Studies of the pathogenesis of interstitial cystitis, obstructive uropathy and intestinal malabsorption in a SLE patient. Am J Med 70:875–881

Williams RC (1981) Immune complexes in human diseases. Ann Rev Med 32:13–28

Chapter 9

Mast Cells and Interstitial Cystitis

F. Aldenborg, M. Fall and L. Enerbäck

Mast cells are widely distributed throughout the connective tissue of most organs. They are numerous in the skin and in mucosal membranes, areas that are exposed to the exterior environment. Mast cells contain potent, pharmacologically active mediators and express plasma membrane receptors with a high affinity to the Fc portion of the IgE antibody (Ishizaka and Ishizaka 1969). The cell is the main tissue repository for histamine, which is stored in cytoplasmic granules together with proteoglycan and several proteins such as neutral proteases, acid hydrolases and chemotactic factors. Upon appropriate immunologic or nonimmunologic stimulation the mast cells release their preformed mediators and also generate and release metabolites of arachiodonic acid (see Katz et al. 1985).

In the light microscope, the cells appear round, oval or elongated and contain a rounded nucleus which is often obscured by an abundance of cytoplasmic granules that stain metachromatically with certain cationic dyes. In the electron microscope the most distinctive mast cell feature is its content of electron-dense granules, which often contain highly characteristic lamellar arrays and whorls or scrolls in humans (see Dvorak et al. 1983).

Mucosal Mast Cells in the Rat

Cationic dye-binding and metachromasia form the basis of the light microscopic recognition of mast cells. However, systematic morphologic, histochemical, biochemical and functional studies of rat mast cells have made it clear that mast cells are diverse (see Enerbäck 1986). Mast cells residing in rat intestinal mucosa are of a specific type, usually referred to as mucosal mast cells (MMCs), which differ from the mast cells of skin and other connective tissue sites, referred to as connective tissue mast cells (CTMCs), MMCs require special conditions of fixation in order to be visualized after staining with cationic dyes such as toluidine blue (Enerbäck 1966a). A very distinctive property of MMCs is their susceptibility to strong aldehyde fixation. The cationic dye-binding of MMCs, in contrast to CTMCs, is thus blocked after fixation in routine 4% formaldehyde solutions. However, this blocking of dye-binding can be reversed after trypsination or prolonged staining times, which suggests that the aldehyde blocking of the cationic dye-binding is caused by a diffusion barrier of protein nature, which is not present in the CTMCs of this species. The concept of mast cell heterogeneity has been further substantiated by the finding that the major glycosaminoglycan of MMCs consists of an oversulfated galactosaminoglycan (Enerbäck et al. 1985), rather than heparin, which is contained in rat skin mast cells (Robinson et al. 1985). MMCs contain considerably less histamine than CTMCs (Enerbäck and Wingren 1980; Befus et al. 1982) and in addition they also contain a distinct neutral protease, referred to as rat mast cell protease II (Woodbury et al. 1978), which differs immunologically from the protease of CTMCs, thus making it possible to distinguish the mast cell subsets by immunohistochemical methods (Gibson and Miller 1986). MMCs are also resistant to the histamine-releasing action of Compound 48/80 and instead show a proliferative response after five days' treatment with this drug (Enerbäck 1966b; Aldenborg 1987).

Studies of the effect of antiallergic drugs acting on mast cells, such as disodium chromoglycate on antigen-specific histamine release by MMCs and CTMCs, have shown that such drugs display a high degree of subset specificity in their action (Bienenstock et al. 1982; Pearce 1986), thus providing pharmacologic, clinically interesting evidence of the diversity of mast cells. MMCs, in contrast to CTMCs, have also proved very sensitive to corticosteroid treatment, but it is not yet known whether this sensitivity is an intrinsic property of the MMC itself or an effect of an interaction with other cells (Miller et al. 1986).

Mucosal Mast Cells in Man

Human mucosal membranes also contain mast cells which differ phenotypically from the mast cells of other tissue sites, but much less is known about their biochemical and functional properties than is the case in the rat. Using several different fixatives, Strobel et al. (1981) found that human intestinal mucosal mast cells were also susceptible to aldehyde fixation, a finding that has been corroborated by other investigators (Ruitenberg et al. 1982; Befus et al. 1985). The requirement of special fixation conditions is therefore also a distinctive property of the human MMC. The extent of aldehyde-induced blocking of the dye-binding of human mast cells has been quantified by the counting of mast cells in optimally fixed tissues before and after formaldehyde treatment (see Enerbäck 1987). The results have shown that mast cells residing in gut and nasal mucosa are blocked to a great extent (80%–90%) by strong aldehyde fixation, while the degree of blocking of mast cells in the skin is of the order of 20%. This implies that mast cell numbers in mucosal membranes may have been grossly underestimated in previous studies, where routine formaldehyde-containing fixatives were used. The properties of the proteoglycan of human MMCs and CTMCs have been further investigated by in situ histochemical methods (see Enerbäck 1987). The results of the chemical and enzymatic degradation of mast cell glycosaminoglycan in situ and the determination of the critical electrolyte concentration of dye-binding (Scott and Dorling, 1965) indicate that human MMCs contain a heparin proteoglycan, but of a different structure than that found in submucosal mast cells and in mast cells of other sites. Recent results have also indicated that human MMCs differ from the mast cells of other sites by their proteinase composition. They can thus be distinguished immuno-histochemically from CTMCs by their predominant content of tryptase, and lack of the chymotryptic proteinase which is the second proteinase of CTCMs (Irani et al. 1986).

Proliferation and Intraepithelial Distribution of MMCs

A distinctive property of MMCs is their strong proliferation in response to infection with the nematode *N. brasiliensis*, located on the surface of the intestinal mucosa during the intestinal phase of the infestation (Miller and Jarrett 1971). The mast cell response is accompanied by a parallel increase in intestinal histamine content and also by the production of both helminth-specific and unspecific IgE antibodies (Jarrett and Miller 1982). MMC-derived specific proteinase (mast cell protease II) is released in high quantities during the infection when mast cells also migrate into the intestinal epithelium; this is indicative of mast cell activation and suggests a functional role for the MMCs during the immune elimination of the nematode (Miller et al. 1986; Woodbury et al. 1984). The mast cell proliferation is immunologically mediated, and is dependent on T lymphocytes (Ruitenberg and Elgersma, 1976). A somewhat similar reaction with numerous mast cells located in the epithelium has been observed in the urinary tract in rats infected with the nematode *Trichosomoides crassicauda* (Kirkman 1950; Ahlquist and Kohonen 1959), and in the intestinal epithelium of patients with the acquired immunodeficiency syndrome (AIDS) infected with cryptosporidia and microsporidia (Dobbins and Weinstein 1985). A redistribution of mast cells from the mucosal stroma into the epithelium has also been observed during the pollen season in patients with strictly seasonal allergic rhinitis due to birch pollen (Enerbäck et al. 1986). The presence of intraepithelial mast cells in mucosal membranes thus appears to be associated with parasite infections or mucosal allergy, conditions which are also characterized by the production of IgE-antibodies. However, a definite evaluation of the significance of this phenomenon requires a systematic study of the presence of intraepithelial mast cells in a great number of inflammatory conditions of mucosal membranes using techniques that adequately preserve the mucosal mast cells.

Mast Cells in Interstitial Cystitis

Interstitial cystitis (Hunner 1915; Hand 1949) is a chronic inflammatory disease of obscure etiology and pathogenesis. No infectious agent which can be incriminated with certainty has hitherto been isolated from patients, which are most often elderly women. Immune responses, however, may be of significance for its pathogenesis, as suggested by the finding of immunoglobulin and complement deposits in the bladder tissue of these patients (see Matilla 1985). The condition is known to be associated with an activation of the mast cell system, as demonstrated by a migration of basophil cells by the skin window technique (Rebuck et al. 1963) and by the finding of increased mast cell density in the urinary bladders (Simmons 1961; Bohne et al. 1962; Smith and Dehner 1972). Morphologic evidence of detrusor mast cell activation, increased tissue histamine content in the urinary bladder and high detrusor mast cell numbers has moreover been reported by Larsen et al. (1982) and Kastrup et al. (1983).

In a current survey aimed at the histochemical characterization of the mast cells in human mucosal membranes under normal and pathologic conditions we recently studied the distribution and properties of the mast cells in the urinary bladders of patients with interstitial cystitis. Tissue samples, which included detrusor muscle, were obtained by transurethral electroresection from the urinary bladders of patients presenting with the classic ulcer disease and patients with a cystoscopically and clinically different presentation, known as early interstitial cystitis (non-ulcer disease) according to Messing and Stamey (1978). Normal bladder tissue from patients with stress urinary incontinence or vesicoureteral reflux was used for comparison. Bladder washings were also analyzed for the presence of mast cells. (Aldenborg et al. 1986; Fall et al. 1987). Tissue samples were fixed in routine 4% formaldehyde (FA) in order to reveal the blocking of specific dye-binding of the mast cells and in a mixture of 0.6% formaldehyde and 0.5% acetic acid (IFAA), which has proved to be the optimum mixture for the preservation of MMCs. The tissue sections were thereafter surveyed for mast cells under the microscope after staining with the cationic dye toluidine blue.

In accordance with other investigators we found that the mast cell density per square unit of detrusor muscle in patients with the classic disease was significantly higher than in the controls. This was particularly so in areas which displayed cystoscopically detectable lesions. The number of mast cells residing in the bladder mucosa or detrusor muscle of controls and patients with non-ulcer disease did not differ significantly, irrespective of the fixation used. Mast cell numbers in the mucosa of specimens obtained from classic lesions were not significantly higher, as compared with the controls, after fixation in FA and staining for 30 min. In contrast, IFAA fixation or prolonged staining resulted in the virtual doubling of the detectable mast cells in the vicinity of classic lesions, thereby indicating that these cells were highly susceptible to aldehyde fixation and not detectable after the use of FA.

Mast cells residing in the lamina propria of controls and the detrusor muscle of all the subjects investigated exhibited approximately the same degree of aldehyde-induced blocking of dye-binding, about 25% (expressed as the fraction of the cells that could not be visualized in FA-fixed tissue after staining for 30 min but after 5 days or after IFAA fixation and staining for 30 min). This blocking of dye-binding was thus of the same magnitude as that of human skin CTMCs (see Enerbäck 1987). On the other hand, the degree of blocking of the mast cells in the mucosal tissue of classic lesions was of the order of 65% (Fig. 9.1), a percentage obviously determined by the population of the bladder mucosa by a subpopulation of completely blocked mast cells in addition to the population of mast cells which is normally found there and in which the blocking

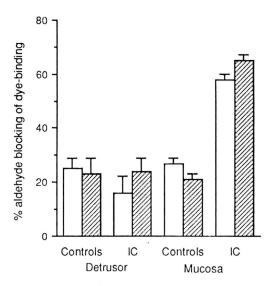

Fig. 9.1. Blocking of dye-binding by aldehyde of mast cells in the detrusor muscle and mucosa in 16 patients with interstitial cystitis and 14 normal control individuals. Mast cells were counted in adjacent tissue sections or in sections of adjacent tissue pieces, and the degree of blocking expressed as the number of cells that could not be visualized in FA-fixed tissue by staining for 30 min but after staining for 5 days (*open bars*) or after IFAA fixation and staining for 30 min (*hatched bars*). Standard errors are indicated by *vertical bars*.

was of the order of 25%.

Patients with the classic disease were also observed to have aldehyde-sensitive mast cells located at all levels of the epithelium (Figs. 9.2, 9.3), while this was not observed in non-ulcer disease or control subjects. The ultrastructure of these intraepithelial mast cells was that of typical human mast cells with rounded nuclei and granules containing lamellar arrays and scrolls. Cytospin preparations were therefore prepared from bladder washings and urine in order to screen for mast cells. We found that both the urine (unpublished observation) and bladder washings of patients with the classic disease contained mast cells which could easily be identified after staining with the cationic dye toluidine blue, while such cells were either absent or very scant in the other patient groups; this is consistent with the histopathologic findings. The number of mast cells in the bladder washings of patients with the classic disease was calculated as ranging between 1000 and 8000 cells per washing. The mast cells thus obtained proved to be extremely well preserved, as judged from their electron microscopic appearance (Fig. 9.4). We therefore measured the histamine content in pellets obtained by the centrifugation of washing fluid, using a sensitive high performance liquid chromatography HPLC technique. Pellets prepared from the bladder washings performed on 16 patients with the classic disease were found to have a histamine content of 18.8±4.3 ng/litre (SEM), determined in total cell pellets obtained by the centrifugation of 1 litre of washing fluid from each patient. The pellet histamine content and mast cell numbers correlated well ($r=$ 0.87) and the calculated histamine content per cell, determined from the mast cell counts and histamine measurements, was found to be 7.6±0.65 pg

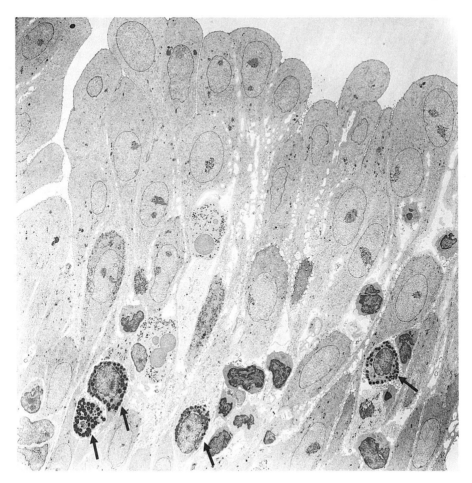

Fig. 9.2. Electron micrograph of intraepithelial mast cells (*arrows*) in a patient with interstitial cystitis. Specimen obtained before distension of the bladder. The mast cells contain many electron-dense granules in the cytoplasm. (×1750)

(Enerbäck et al. 1989). This histamine content is higher than the 2.8 pg/cell reported in mast cells isolated from chopped and enzymatically treated human intestinal tissue (Fox et al. 1985), but of the same order as that calculated for mast cells in nasal lavage preparations from allergic subjects (Pipkorn et al. 1989). The discrepancy may reflect that the mast cells obtained by the bladder washings or by nasal lavage were never subjected to potential histamine-releasing procedures, hitherto one of the only ways of obtaining human mast cells in suspension. The protocol used for the mast cell quantification and histamine measurements is shown below:

Mast Cells and Histamine in Bladder Washings:
Flush 1 litre of cystoscopy fluid (aminoacetic acid, 22 mg/ml in distilled water, pH 6), divided into portions of approximately 50 ml, gently into the undistended bladder and recover the fluid.

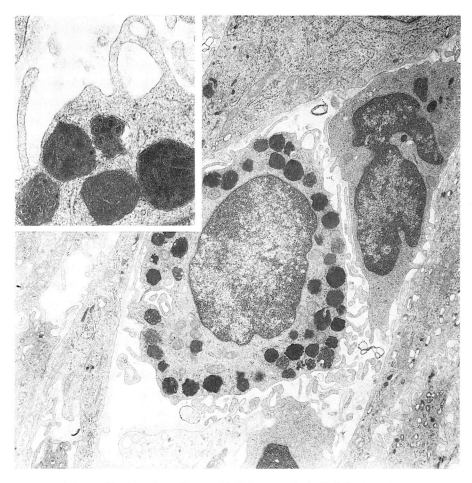

Fig. 9.3. High-magnification view of intraepithelial mast cell. (×10 500). *Inset* shows mast cell granules containing typical scrolls. (×37 000)

Cool the recovered fluid on ice and centrifuge at 250 *g* for 5 min.

Resuspend pellet in 1–3 ml Hank's balanced salt solution containing 0.1% serum albumin.

Mast cells:

Centrifuge 50 *μ*l samples of the resuspended pellet on object slides using a cytocentrifuge (Shandon Cytospin, 1500 rpm for 5 min).

Air-dry (15 min), fix in methanol (10 min), and stain with 0.5% toluidine blue dissolved in 0.5% HCl (30 min).

Dehydrate and mount under coverslips in a synthetic resin.

Count total number of mast cells per specimen.

Histamine:

Centrifuge at 250 *g* for 5 min.

Discard supernatant, add 250–500 *μ*l 0.4% $HClO_4$ and shake with a Vortex mixer.

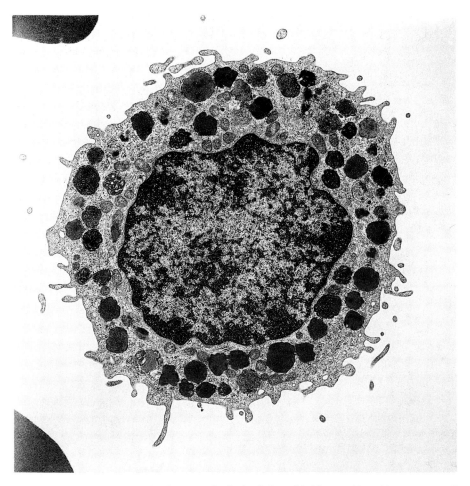

Fig. 9.4. Electron micrograph of mast cell obtained from bladder washing. Note many well-preserved electron-dense granules. ($\times 13\ 500$)

Adjust to pH 6.5 by adding 5 M K_2CO_3 using bromphenol blue as an indicator, and centrifuge at 4000 g for 15 min to remove precipitated $KClO_4$.

Filter the clear supernatant through a Durapore 0.45 μm membrane filter (Millipore Corp.) and measure histamine using an HPLC-assay.

The mast cells in the urinary bladders of patients with classic interstitial cystitis have been further characterized using in situ histochemical techniques (Aldenborg et al. unpublished data). In addition to the previous finding of a high degree of aldehyde blocking of the mast cells in the bladder mucosa, we have found that the mast cells obtained by bladder washings and the mast cells residing in bladder mucosa exhibited a lower critical electrolyte concentration of dye-binding than the mast cells residing in detrusor musculature, thus reflecting differences in the charge density and/or molecular size of their glycosaminoglycans. Enzymatic degradation with chondroitinase did not abolish the cationic dye-binding of either detrusor or lamina propria mast cells.

However, this was abolished after the specific degradation of heparin with nitrous acid (Shively and Conrad 1976), thus suggesting that all the mast cells in the urinary bladder and in bladder washings contain a heparin proteoglycan, but of a different structure depending on the tissue site.

The accumulated results thus provide firm evidence of the expansion of two different mast cell subsets in the urinary bladders of patients with classic interstitial cystitis. Mast cells with the phenotypic appearance of CTMC are found in high numbers in the detrusor musculature and mast cells, which phenotypically appear as MMCs of other mucosal sites, greatly increase in number in the bladder mucosa in the vicinity of classic lesions.

Implications

The presence of intraepithelial mast cells is a rare event under normal physiologic circumstances, but is a characteristic finding under certain pathologic conditions where the IgE system is involved. Our findings of a local recruitment and transepithelial migration of mast cells along with the previous observation of a migration of mast cells or basophils using the skin window technique (Rebuck et al. 1963) in patients with classic interstitial cystitis provide evidence of a functional activation of the mast cell system in this disease entity.

The diagnosis of classic interstitial cystitis is based on the clinical presentation, cystoscopic observations and histopathologic findings. The finding of detrusor and mucosal mast cell hyperplasia and intraepithelial mast cells and mast cells in bladder washings is useful when establishing the diagnosis. These observations have also proved to be of value for distinguishing the classic disease from so-called early interstitial cystitis in which there are no signs of mast cell activation (Fall et al. 1987). The finding of mast cells and histamine in pellets obtained from the bladder washings of patients with the classic disease may serve as a useful tool for establishing the diagnosis under circumstances where surgical biopsies cannot easily be obtained, such as in outpatient departments. The histamine and mast cell content in individual washings from the same patient are potentially useful indicators of the disease activity. In our experience the severity of symptoms and lesions observed at cystoscopy thus seems to be fairly well correlated with these parameters.

Mast cells are secretory cells which can be stimulated to secretion through the binding of an appropriate antigen to their IgE surface receptors. Mast cell secretion can also be induced by many nonimmunologic agents such as Compound 48/80, lectins and calcium ionophores (see Lagunoff et al. 1983). It has recently become clear that mast cell secretion can also be induced by neurotransmitters such as substance P, which releases histamine from both MMCs and CTMCs (Shanahan et al. 1985). Sensory nerve fibres containing substance P have been found both in the bladder wall and in the epithelium of rat urinary bladders (Yokokawa et al. 1985). These findings are of great interest, since evidence has been presented which suggests a direct innervation of mast cells (Newson et al. 1983). Local immune responses can therefore also be modulated by peripheral sensory nerve activity.

Some of the symptoms and findings in interstitial cystitis, such as frequency and pain and mucosal edema observed at cystoscopy, may be related to the release of preformed or secondarily generated mast cell mediators. Histamine can thus cause the contraction of smooth muscle and increased vascular permeability, leading to edema, and arachidonic acid metabolites can cause pain and initiate a multitude of complex inflammatory events where inflammatory cells, attracted by mast-cell-derived chemotactic factors, participate. The prolonged inflammatory response in interstitial cystitis may also be the result of mast cell stimulation. Allergen challenge can thus give rise to a late phase inflammatory reaction characterized by the infiltration of the tissue of lymphocytes, eosinophils and neutrophils. The reaction seems to be IgE-dependent and may also be mediated by mast cells (Dolovich et al. 1973; Solley et al. 1976). This late phase reaction may appear to be a link between allergen challenge and continuous inflammatory allergic disease. Mast-cell-derived factors also appear to interact with fibroblasts. This may be taken as indirect evidence of a role of the mast cells in tissue repair and fibrosis (Norrby et al. 1976; Franzén and Norrby 1982; Atkins et al. 1985).

The mast cell hyperplasia and intraepithelial migration of MMCs in interstitial cystitis is reminiscent of the mast cell reaction observed in animal nematode models or in nasal allergic conditions. This suggests that the mast cell-IgE system may be of significance for the pathogenesis of classic interstitial cystitis. The mast cell accumulation can be the result of the local proliferation of differentiated cells (Enerbäck and Rundquist 1981; Sonoda et al. 1984), be due to the proliferation of committed fixed tissue precursors (Matsuda et al. 1981) or involve the homing and proliferation of bone-marrow-derived circulating progenitors (Kitamura et al. 1979; Zucker-Franklin et al. 1981).

The nature of the factors which are responsible for the hyperplasia and migration of mast cells in interstitial cystitis are unknown. However, the finding of mast cell activation in this disease implies that we should reconsider the possibility of a parasitic infection involving a hitherto unrecognized microorganism, as well as a parasitic allergy or an allergic reaction to a nonparasitic allergen located in the bladder tissue or the urine, being involved in the etiology of the disease.

References

Ahlquist J, Kohonen J (1959) On the granulated cells of the urinary tract in rats infected with *Trichosomoides crassicauda*. Acta Pathol Microbiol Scand 46:313–319

Aldenborg, F (1987) Thymus dependence of Compound 48/80-induced mucosal mast cell proliferation. Int Arch Allergy Appl Immunol 84:298–305

Aldenborg F, Fall M, Enerbäck L (1986) Proliferation and transepithelial migration of mucosal mast cells in interstitial cystits. Immunology 58:411–416

Atkins FM, Friedman MM, Pillarisetti VSF, Metcalfe DD (1985) Interactions between mast cells, fibroblasts and connective tissue components. Int Arch Allergy Appl Immunol 77:96–102

Befus AD, Pearce FL, Gauldie J, Horsewood P, Bienenstock J (1982) Mucosal mast cells. I. Isolation and functional characteristics of rat intestinal mast cells. J Immunol 128:2475–2480

Befus AD, Goodacre R, Dyck N, Bienenstock J (1985) Mast cell heterogeneity in man. I. Histologic studies of the intestine. Int Arch Allergy Appl Immunol 76:232–236

Bienenstock J, Befus AD, Pearce F, Denburg J, Goodacre R (1982) Mast cell heterogeneity: derivation and function, with emphasis on the intestine. J Allergy Clin Immunol 70:407–412

Bohne AW, Hodson JM, Rebuck JW, Reinhard RE (1962) An abnormal leukocyte response in interstitial cystitis. J Urol 88:387–391

Dobbins WO III, Weinstein WM (1985) Electron microscopy of the intestine and rectum in acquired immunodeficiency syndrome. Gastroenterology 88:738–749

Dolovich J, Hargreave FE, Chalmers R, Shier KJ, Gauldie J, Bienenstock J (1973) Late cutaneous allergic responses in isolated IgE-dependent reactions. J Allergy Clin Immunol 52:38–46

Dvorak AM, Dvorak HF, Galli SJ (1983) Ultrastructural criteria for identification of mast cells and basophils in humans, guinea pigs, and mice. Am Rev Respir Dis 128:49–52

Enerbäck L (1966a) Mast cells in rat gastrointestinal mucosa. II. Dye-binding and metachromatic properties. Acta Pathol Microbiol Scand 66:303–312

Enerbäck L (1966b) Mast cells in rat gastrointestinal mucosa. III. Reactivity towards Compound 48/80. Acta Pathol Microbiol Scand 66:313–322

Enerbäck L (1986) Mast cell heterogeneity: the evolution of the concept of a specific mucosal mast cell. In: Befus AD, Bienenstock J, Denburg J (eds) Mast cell differentiation and heterogeneity. Raven, New York pp 1–26

Enerbäck L (1987) Mucosal mast cells in the rat and in man. Int Arch Allergy Appl Immunol 82:249–255

Enerbäck L, Rundquist I (1981) DNA distribution of mast cell populations in growing rats. Histochemistry 71:521–531

Enerbäck L, Wingren U (1980) Histamine content of peritoneal and tissue mast cells of growing rats. Histochemistry 66:113–124

Enerbäck L, Kolset SO, Kusche M, Hjerpe A, Lindahl U (1985) Glycosaminoglycans in rat mucosal mast cells. Biochem J 227:661–668

Enerbäck L, Pipkorn U, Granerus G (1986) Intraepithelial migration of nasal mucosal mast cells in hay fever. Int Arch Allergy Appl Immunol 80:44–51

Enerbäck L, Fall M, Aldenborg F (1989) Histamine and mucosal mast cells in interstitial cystitis. Agents Actions 26:113–116

Fall M, Johansson SL, Aldenborg F (1987) Chronic interstitial cystitis: a heterogeneous syndrome. J Urol 137:35–38

Fox CC, Dvorak AM, Peters SP, Kagey-Sobotka A, Lichtenstein LM (1985) Isolation and characterization of human intestinal mucosal mast cells. J Immunol 135:483–491

Franzén L, Norrby K (1982) Immunological challenge causes mitogenic stimulation in normal connective tissue cells. Acta Pathol Microbiol Immunol Scand [A] 90:385–389

Gibson S, Miller HRP (1986) Mast cell subsets in the rat distinguished immunohistochemically by their content of serine proteinases. Immunology 58:101–104

Hand JR (1949) Interstitial cystitis: report of 223 cases (204 women and 19 men). J Urol 61:291–310

Hunner GL (1915) A rare type of bladder ulcer in women: report of cases. Boston Med Surg J 172:660–662

Irani AA, Schechter NM, Craig SS, DeBlois G, Schwartz LB (1986) Two types of human mast cells that have distinct neutral protease composition. Proc Natl Acad Sci USA 83:4464–4468

Ishizaka K, Ishizaka T (1969) Immune mechanism of reversed type reaginic hypersensitivity. J Immunol 103:588–595

Jarrett EEE, Miller HRP (1982) Production and activities of IgE in helminth infection. Prog Allergy 31:178–233

Kastrup J, Hald T, Larsen S, Nielsen VG (1983) Histamine content and mast cell count of detrusor muscle in patients with interstitial cystitis and other types of chronic cystitis. Br J Urol 55:495–500

Katz HR, Stevens RL, Austen KF (1985) Leukotriene and prostaglandin pathway metabolism. Heterogeneity of mammalian mast cells differentiated in vivo and in vitro. J Allergy Clin Immunol 76:250–259

Kirkman H (1950) A comparative morphological and cytochemical study of globule leucocytes (Schollenleukocyten) of the urinary tract and of possibly related cells. Am J Anat 86:91–130

Kitamura Y, Hatanaka K, Murakami M, Shibata H (1979) Presence of mast cell precursors in peripheral blood of mice demonstrated by parabiosis. Blood 53:1085–1088

Lagunoff D, Martin TW, Read G (1983) Agents that release histamine from mast cells. Annu Rev Pharmacol Toxicol 23:331–351

Larsen S, Thomson SA, Hald T et al. (1982) Mast cells in interstitial cystitis. Br J Urol 54:283–286

Matsuda H, Kitamura Y, Sonoda T, Imori T (1981) Precursor of mast cells fixed in the skin of mice. J Cell Physiol 108:409–415

Mattila J (1985) Immunopathology of interstitial cystitis. Dissertation. Acta Universitatis Tamperensis, ser A vol 184

Messing EM, Stamey TA (1978) Interstitial cystitis. Early diagnosis, pathology, and treatment. Urology 12:381–392

Miller HRP, Jarrett WHF (1971) Immune reactions in mucous membranes. I. Intestinal mast cell response during helminth expulsion in the rat. Immunology 20:277–288

Miller HRP, King SJ, Gibson S, Huntley JF, Newlands GFJ, Woodbury RG (1986) Intestinal mucosal mast cells in normal and parasitized rats. In: Befus AD, Bienenstock J, Denburg J (eds) Mast cell differentiation and heterogeneity. Raven, New York pp 239–255

Newson B, Dahlström A, Enerbäck L, Ahlman H (1983) Suggestive evidence for a direct innervation of mucosal mast cells. Neuroscience 10:565–570

Norrby K, Enerbäck L, Franzén L (1976) Mast cell activation and tissue cell proliferation. Cell Tissue Res 30 170:289–303

Pearce FL (1986) On the heterogeneity of mast cells. Pharmacology 32:61–71

Pipkorn U, Karlsson G, Enerbäck L (1989) Nasal mucosal response to repeated challenges with pollen allergen. Am Rev Resp Dis 140:729–736

Rebuck JW, Hodson JM, Priest RJ, Barth CL (1963) Basophilic granulocytes in inflammatory tissues of man. Ann NY Acad Sci 103:409–425

Robinson HC, Horner AA, Höök M, Ögren S, Lindahl U (1978) A proteoglycan form of heparin and its degradation to single-chain molecules. J Biol Chem 253:6687–6693

Ruitenberg EJ, Elgersma A (1976) Absence of intestinal mast cell response in congenitally athymic mice during *Trichinella spiralis* infection. Nature 264:258–260

Ruitenberg EJ, Gustowska L, Elgersma A, Ruitenberg HM (1982) Effect of fixation on the light microscopical visualization of mast cells in the mucosa and connective tissue of the human duodenum. Int Arch Allergy Appl Immunol 67:233–238

Scott JE, Dorling J (1965) Differential staining of acid glycosaminoglycans (mucopolysaccharides) by alcian blue in salt solutions. Histochemie 5:221–233

Shanahan F, Denburg JA, Fox J, Bienenstock J, Befus DA (1985) Mast cell heterogenity: effects of neuroenteric peptides on histamine release. J Immunol 135:1331–1337

Shively JE, Conrad HE (1976) Formation of anhydrosugars in the chemical depolymerization of heparin. Biochemistry 15:3932–3942

Simmons JI (1961) Interstitial cystitis: an explanation for the beneficial effect of an antihistamine. J Urology 85:149–155

Smith BH, Dehner LP (1972) Chronic ulcerating interstitial cystitis (Hunner's ulcer). A study of 28 cases. Arch Pathol 93:76–81

Solley GO, Gleich GJ, Jordon RE, Schroeter AL (1976) The late phase of the immediate weal and flare skin reaction. Its dependence upon IgE antibodies. J Clin Invest 58:408–420

Sonoda T, Kanayama Y, Hara H et al. (1984) Proliferation of peritoneal mast cells in the skin of W/W^v mice that genetically lack mast cells. J. Exp Med 160:138–151

Strobel S, Miller HRP, Ferguson A (1981) Human intestinal mucosal mast cells. Evaluation of fixation and staining techniques. J Clin Pathol 34:851–858

Woodbury R, Gruzenski GM, Lagunoff D (1978) Immunofluorescent localization of a serine protease in rat small intestine. Proc Natl Acad Sci USA 75:2785–2789

Woodbury RG, Miller HRP, Huntley JF, Newlands GFJ, Palliser AC, Wakelin D (1989) Mucosal mast cells are functionally active during spontaneous expulsion of intestinal nematode infections in rat. Nature 312:450–452

Yokokawa K, Sakanaka M, Shiosaka S, Tohyama M, Shiotani Y, Sonoda T (1985) Three-dimensional distribution of substance P-like immunoreactivity in the urinary bladder of rat. J Neural Transm 63:209–222

Zucker-Franklin D, Grusky G, Hirayama N, Schnipper E (1981) The presence of mast cell precursors in rat peripheral blood. Blood 58:544–551

Chapter 10

Diagnosis of Interstitial Cystitis: A Clinical, Endoscopic and Pathologic Approach

G.R. Sant

Interstitial cystitis (IC) is frequently a diagnosis of exclusion in patients with irritative voiding symptons and negative urine cultures. The true incidence of IC is difficult to ascertain because of non-uniform clinical, endoscopic and histologic diagnostic criteria (Sant 1987). Oravisto estimated the incidence of IC in Finland to be 18 per 100 000 women (Oravisto 1975). However, a recent questionnaire survey estimated the prevalence of IC in the United States to be at least twice that in Finland (Held et al. 1987). Females are affected ten times more frequently than men. The condition is not common in blacks, children or adolescents (Geist and Antolak 1970).

The clinical course of IC is frequently punctuated by periods of exacerbation and remission and spontaneous remission has been reported in 10%–15% of cases (Oravisto 1975: Messing and Stamey 1978). Although about 10% of the patients have "classic" Hunner's disease with mucosal ulcers and reduced bladder capacities (Hunner 1915), the vast majority have non-ulcerated bladders of normal or slightly subnormal capacity (Messing and Stamey 1978; Webster and Galloway 1987).

The "classic" variety of IC described by Hunner usually occurs in middle-aged and older women and is more prevalent in Europe, accounting for over half of the patients in a recent report (Fall et al. 1987). This "ulcer" type of IC is distinctly uncommon in the USA, accounting for less than 5%–10% of cases (Webster and Galloway 1987; Meares Jr 1987). IC most commonly affects young women and they have a normal bladder capacity and an absence of bladder fibrosis or ulcers. The variable natural history of IC begets the question as to whether the "early" form of IC described by Messing and Stamey (1978) inexorably progresses to the "classic" form. The two clinical forms of the disease may well have differing etiology and pathogenesis or they may represent opposite ends of a disease spectrum. It has been suggested that interstitial cystitis is a bladder symptom complex of multifactorial etiology (Fall et al. 1987).

Symptomatology

Irritative voiding symptoms such as frequency, urgency and nocturia are common in IC. Suprapubic and/or pelvic pain is usually prominent. The pain is typically related to bladder filling and relieved by voiding, although some patients complain of pain at the end of voiding. Fixed suprapubic pain and dyspareunia are common. Dysuria and incontinence rarely occur.

Abdomino-pelvic examination is usually normal although deep suprapubic tenderness on palpation or anterior vaginal wall tenderness in the region of the bladder trigone can be present in some patients. Neurologic examination is normal. A careful gynecologic examination excludes conditions which can give rise to the same symptoms as IC such as vaginitis, urethral diverticula and vestibular adenitis. Many female patients with IC have undergone prior gynecologic surgery such as hysterectomy or laparoscopy, or experience worsening of their symptoms at the time of their monthly menses. Males comprise 10% of IC patients (Messing and Stamey 1978). They complain of perineal, scrotal or groin discomfort – symptoms suggestive of the "prostatitis syndrome". Bacterial localization cultures (VB_1, VB_2, EPS and VC_3) and microscopic examination of expressed prostatic secretions (EPS) should be done to identify patients with chronic bacterial and non-bacterial prostatitis. Prostatodynia patients may have the endoscopic features of "early" IC when cystoscoped under anaesthesia (Messing 1987) and this suggests that a sub-group of male patients with IC may well have prostatodynia.

Diagnosis

The diagnosis of IC requires a high index of clinical suspicion (Table 10.1). Patients with symptoms of vesical irritability and pain who have negative cultures should be suspected of having IC. Pyuria in a patient with a negative midstream urine culture may be indicative of the "urethral syndrome". Quantitative urine cultures should be done to identify patients with "low count" bacteriuria (colony counts less than 10^5 bacteria per ml of urine), who require oral antimicrobial therapy. Non-bacteriuric patients with pyuria should have

Table 10.1. Diagnostic considerations

High index of clinical suspicion
Exclude
"classic" bacteriuria ($>10^5$ bacteria/ml)
"low count" bacteriuria ($<10^5$ bacteria/ml)
carcinoma in situ
mucosal dysplasia
specific cystitis (tuberculous, radiation, etc.)
prostatitis syndromes
Urodynamic evaluation in selected patients
Gynecologic assessment

cultures performed to exclude chlamydial infection. Pyuria and hematuria are uncommon although about 10% of patients have > 10 white blood cells or > 5 red blood cells per high power field (Messing 1987). Gross, painless hematuria is an occasional presenting feature of IC. The diagnosis of IC cannot be made in the presence of bacterial cystitis. A prior history of cystitis does not exclude the diagnosis of IC if the patient continues to be symptomatic in spite of a sterile urine. Some patients report the onset of their symptoms following a course of antibiotic treatment for documented bacterial urinary tract infections.

Carcinoma in situ (CIS) and bladder mucosal dysplasia cause irritative voiding symptoms and their cystoscopic appearances can be similar to those of IC. Carcinoma in situ was present in 23% of men referred for evaluation of interstitial cystitis to the Mayo Clinic (Utz and Zincke 1974). A negative urine cytology or bladder biopsy is required, especially in male patients, before a diagnosis of interstitial cystitis can be made (Utz and Zincke 1974; Meares Jr 1987).

Video-urodynamic studies are not diagnostic of IC. Urodynamic investigation is often uncomfortable because of severe sensory urgency and suprapubic discomfort during bladder filling. Most IC patients have stable detrusors and normal bladder compliance. Patients with significant incontinence or lack of pain, benefit from urodynamic evaluation to assess vesicourethral function (Perez-Marrero et al. 1987). Detrusor instability occurs in a small percentage of IC patients and requires further evaluation to exclude a neurologic etiology (Holm-Bentzen et al. 1987a). Urodynamic testing is also helpful in monitoring response to therapy and in the selection of patients for surgical cystoplasty procedures (Webster and Galloway 1987).

Radiographic imaging will diagnose conditions such as tuberculous cystitis or bladder calculi that may be confused with IC. Patients with severely reduced bladder capacities may have upper tract dilatation secondary to ureterovesical junction (UVJ) obstruction. Voiding cystourethrograms (VCUGs) are not routinely indicated although patients with small bladders due to eosinophilic or tuberculous cystitis may have vesicoureteral reflux (VUR).

There is no consensus regarding the use of laboratory tests (e.g. antinuclear antibody titers) for the diagnosis of IC. Assay of urinary histamine metabolites, epidermal growth factor, prostaglandins, glycosaminoglycans (GAGs) and eosinophilic cationic protein (ECP) have not yet been applied to the routine, non-invasive, clinical diagnosis of IC (Messing 1987; Lose et al. 1987; Holm-Bentzen et al. 1987b).

Cystoscopy is widely regarded as a prerequisite for the diagnosis of IC and should be done under general or spinal anaesthesia (Table 10.2). The presence of "glomerulations" is regarded as one of the endoscopic hallmarks of the disease and they appear as diffuse, small, submucosal, petechial hemorrhages after the bladder is filled to capacity (Messing and Stamey 1978). Although highly suggestive. "glomerulations" are not pathognomonic of IC. They may occur in tuberculous cystitis, cyclophosphamide-induced cystitis, radiation cystitis, distension of a defunctionalized bladder and carcinoma in situ. We have also noted it in patients who have received intravesical thiotepa chemotherapy for treatment of recurrent superficial bladder tumors. Cystoscopy performed under local anaesthesia may not reveal the presence or the true extent of "glomerulations". Bladder capacity is measured by passive gravity filling of the bladder with the irrigating fluid held at a hydrostatic pressure of 70–80 cm H_2O

Table 10.2. Interstitial cystitis: endoscopic considerations

Cystoscopy under anesthesia
Normal urethral lamen
"Glomerulations"
Terminal "blood-tinge"
"Early" disease
  capacity > 400 ml
  no ulcers, scars
"Classic" disease
  capacity < 400 ml
  ulcers, scars
Biopsy to exclude specific disease

---

for about 1 minute. The bladder should not be "hydrodilated" by syringe-filling or by prolonging filling after the bladder capacity is reached. Filling measures the true as opposed to the functional bladder capacity. Drainage of the bladder after it is filled to capacity usually results in a terminal blood-tinge of the draining fluid secondary to oozing from the areas of "glomerulation". Such bleeding, especially after a second filling, occurs in about 90% of patients (Messing and Stamey 1978; Holm-Bentzen et al. 1987a). The typical patient with "early" IC is a young to middle-aged woman with a normal or near-normal bladder capacity under anaesthesia, "glomerulations" on bladder filling and terminal bleeding on drainage of the irrigation fluid (Meares Jr 1987).

"Glomerulations" and bleeding may not be fully appreciated until the bladder is filled to capacity for a second time. The changes typically involve the dome, posterior and lateral walls of the bladder and spares the trigone. The cystoscopic findings frequently do not parallel the type or severity of symptoms or the subsequent response to treatment (Messing 1987). Urethral calibration is usually normal and urethral dilatation is seldom indicated. Hunner's ulcer and/or a reduced bladder are infrequently seen because most patients suffer from the "early" or "non-ulcer" variety of IC. Hunner's ulcer is, therefore, not a requirement for the diagnosis of IC. This is not widely appreciated and may result in misdiagnosis in patients who do not have bladder ulcers (Meares Jr 1987; Messing 1987). The "classic" form of IC is characterized by a bladder capacity of less than 350–400 ml under anaesthesia and the presence of fissures and scars which tend to split and bleed as capacity is approached (Webster and Galloway 1987).

Pathologic Features

Interstitial cystitis is characterized pathologically by a non-specific chronic inflammatory infiltrate, edema and vasodilatation of the submucosa and detrusor layers of the bladder wall (Smith and Dehner 1972; Holm-Bentzen et al. 1985). The histologic changes are diffuse and reflect neither the endoscopic findings, the severity or the duration of symptoms. Patients with "classic" IC are more likely to have inflammation and fibrosis of the detrusor muscle. Biopsy not only confirms bladder wall ("interstitial") inflammation ("cystitis") but serves to exclude specific diseases such as carcinoma in situ, eosinophilic cystitis or tuberculous cystitis. The specimen should include mucosa and underlying muscle so as to provide an adequate sample for the assessment of both submucosal and detrusor inflammation ("pancystitis"). Biopsies can be safely obtained using cup-biopsy forceps after the cystoscopy and bladder filling maneuvers. Bladder perforation is rare if the biopsy is obtained from the lateral bladder wall with the bladder almost empty. Two biopsies (one from each lateral wall) usually provide adequate tissue for pathologic examination. Transurethral biopsies are recommended by some European authors (Fall et al. 1987) but this increases the likelihood of bladder perforation and post-biopsy morbidity. Cystoscopy and "deep" bladder biopsy can usually be carried out in the day-surgery or ambulatory surgery suite and, in this setting, cup-biopsies are safer than transurethral biopsies. The pathologic changes in the bladder are diffuse and the specimens obtained with the cup-biopsy forceps are adequate for histologic assessment of bladder inflammation. Perineural inflammation, eosinophilic leukocyte infiltrate and detrusor fibrosis are infrequently encountered in patients with the "early" form of interstitial cystitis (Holm-Bentzen and Lose 1987). Following the biopsy (mucosa and muscle) procedure, the bladder should be drained with a Foley catheter for 24 h.

Bladder biopsy will exclude specific disease entities and confirm the presence of bladder wall inflammation ("interstitial cystitis"). Although some authors claim that biopsy is not routinely required for diagnosis, the biopsy material is useful for investigative study and it may help categorize sub-groups of patients based on specific histologic criteria. Such "histopathologic typing" may hopefully allow tailored approaches to diagnosis and treatment.

Bladder "Mastocytosis"

Many studies have noted the presence of a mast cell infiltrate in the bladder wall of patients with IC (Larsen et al. 1982; Feltis, et al. 1987; Lynes et al. 1987) suggesting a potential pathogenetic role of the mast cell. Mast cells release potent, pharmacologically active mediators such as histamine, prostaglandins, leukotrienes and tryptases upon exposure to specific antigens and these mediators have significant biologic effects on smooth muscle, vascular epithelium and inflammation (Galli et al. 1984). Mast cells are widely distributed in connective tissues and beneath epithelial surfaces (respiratory, gastrointestinal) and increased numbers of mast cells occur in many diseases, e.g. asthma, coronary artery spasm, celiac disease and rheumatoid arthritis (Estensen 1985; Gruber et al. 1986).

Histamine release was suggested as a cause of the symptoms of IC in the 1950s (Simmons and Bunce 1958). Histamine causes pain, erythema, vasodilatation and fibrosis – features characteristic of IC. Larsen and colleagues suggested a count of > 28 mast cells per mm^2 in the detrusor muscle ("detrusor mastocytosis") as being pathognomic of IC (Larsen et al. 1982). However, a later study by the same group revealed that only 30% (43 out of 115) of a large group of patients with clinical and cystoscopic features suggestive of IC actually

Table 10.3. Bladder mastocytosis in interstitial cystitis

Occurs in 30%–50% patients

Not pathognomic

Ill-defined diagnostic criteria
  staining technique
  role degranulated cells
  mucosal vs tissue cells
  mast cells in other bladder disease

---

had "detrusor mastocytosis" (Holm-Bentzen et al. 1987a). An increase in mast cells has also been demonstrated in the submucosa of patients with the "classic" or "ulcer" variety of interstitial cystitis (Aldenborg et al. 1986). "Mucosal" mast cells were present in the lamina propria and the superficial layers of the transitional epithelium and their recovery from bladder washings was suggested as a new approach to diagnosis. "Mucosal" mast cells, unlike their detrusor or "tissue" counterparts, are susceptible to aldehyde fixation and they require special fixation and staining for their identification. This precludes their routine use in surgical pathology laboratories. The "mucosal" cell differs from the "tissue" cell in staining characteristics, low histamine content, types of proteoglycans and response to histamine liberators and oral antihistamines. The two populations of mast cells were increased in most patients with "classic" IC but there was no statistically significant increase in patients with the "early" variant of the disease (Aldenborg et al. 1986). Other studies, however, have demonstrated increased numbers of mucosal mast cells in patients with "non-ulcer" interstitial cystitis (Feltis et al. 1987; Lynes et al. 1987). Whether the mast cell is just a histologic marker or the pathognomonic feature of interstitial cystitis is unknown (Table 10.3). The mast cell count in the "normal" bladder wall needs to be determined and the mast cell infiltrate in diseases other than interstitial cystitis requires further study. Studies utilizing specialized staining and fixation techniques and the use of a variety of patient controls will determine the mast cell response in conditions such as UTIs and cancer and help to establish numerical criteria (cells per HPF or cells per mm^2) for the diagnosis of "mast cell cystitis".

  Giemsa and toluidine blue stains identify mast cells by virtue of the staining of their cytoplasmic granules. However, partially or fully degranulated mast cells are not reliably identified using these stains. A recent study showed that IC patients had more detrusor mast cells (granulated and degranulated) than controls and the difference was more statistically significant for the degranulated cells (Lynes et al. 1987). The number of degranulated mast cells in the detrusor correlated with the degree of inflammation, ulceration and response to treatment. There was no statistical difference in submucosal mast cell densities between interstitial cystitis (22 patients – 14 with "early" disease, 8 with decreased bladder capacity) and control patients. The average number of detrusor mast cells in IC patients was 57 cells/mm^2 and over half (56%) were degranulated. This study suggests that degranulated mast cells account for a significant proportion of the mast cell infiltrate in IC. Such activated mast cells lose their histologically identifiable granules upon stimulation and degranulation and routine histologic techniques will underestimate their presence in patients with active disease.

The role of the mast cell (granulated and degranulated) requires further study using techniques such as specific IgE mast cell receptor stains and measurement of urinary levels of known mast cell mediators and enzymes, e.g. histamine, prostaglandins and the tryptases. The mast cell is not ubiquitous in the bladder wall of IC patients and mastocytosis is present in only 30%–50% of IC patients (Holm-Bentzen et al. 1987a; Lynes et al. 1987). "Mastocytosis" may well define a sub-group of patients with specific pathogenesis and treatment potential. However, it has not been clearly defined pathologically and the definition of > 28 mast cells/mm^2 does not include degranulated or "mucosal" mast cells (Larsen et al. 1982). The pathogenetic and pathognomonic role of the mast cell in interstitial cystitis remains intriguing. However, an absence of bladder mastocytosis does not exclude the diagnosis of interstitial cystitis. Mast cell quantitation is still largely a research tool and many patients with interstitial cystitis do not have demonstrable increases in mast cell density using conventional histopathologic staining techniques.

Measurement of biologically active mast cell mediators in the urine holds promise as a non-invasive tool for the diagnosis of IC. Increased urinary levels of 1,4-methylimidazole acetic acid (1,4-MIAA), a histamine metabolite, increased concentration of histamine in the bladder wall and elevated urinary prostaglandin E levels have all been demonstrated in patients with "detrusor mastocytosis" (Lose et al. 1987; Holm-Bentzen et al. 1987b). However, urinary assay of these chemicals has not been translated into routine clinical use.

Summary

Interstitial cystitis is a disease that is often puzzling to clinicians. The increase in newly diagnosed cases in recent years is due to better recognition of the disease as well as a rising prevalence of the disease, especially in young and middle-aged females. The wider appreciation of the existence of two clinical varieties of IC – the "early" ("non-ulcer") and the "late" ("classic" or "ulcer") – has led to increased recognition and diagnosis of the condition.

Variation in symptomatology, endoscopic findings, histopathology and response to treatment, suggests that IC may not be one disease but rather a syndrome of heterogenous causation. Identification of these causes should lead to the use of specific treatment modalities and translate into better treatment outcomes for IC patients. The role of the mast cell in IC requires further study and bladder "mastocytosis" needs to be more accurately defined and quantitated.

References

Aldenborg F, Fall M, Enerback L (1986) Proliferation and transepithelial migration of mucosal mast cells in interstitial cystitis. Immunology 58:411–416

Estensen RD (1985) What is the role of myocardial mast cells? Hum Pathol 16:536–538

Fall M, Johannson SL, Aldenborg F (1987) Chronic interstitial cystitis: a heterogenous syndrome. J Urol 137:35–38

Feltis JT, Perez-Marrero R, Emerson LE (1987) Increased mast cells of bladder in suspected cases of interstitial cystitis: possible disease marker. J Urol 138:42–43

Galli SJ, Dvorak AM, Dvorak HF (1984) Basophils and mast cells: morphologic insights into their biology, secretory patterns and function. Prog Allergy 34:1–141

Geist RW, Antolak SJ (1970) Interstitial cystitis in children. J Urol 104:922–925

Gruber B, Poznansky M, Boss E, Partin J, Gorevic P, Kaplan AP (1986) Characterization and functional studies of rheumatoid synovial mast cells. Arthritis Rheum 29:944–955

Held P, Hanno P, Wein A, Pauly M (1987) Epidemiology of interstitial cystitis: incidence of interstitial cystitis from a national sample of urologists. NIDDK Workshop on Interstitial Cystitis, Bethesda, Maryland, August 28–29, 1987

Holm-Bentzen M, Lose G (1987) Pathology and pathogenesis of interstitial cystitis, Urology [Suppl] 29(4):8–13

Holm-Bentzen M, Larsen S, Hainau B, Hald T (1985) Non-obstructive detrusor myopathy in a group of patients with chronic abacterial cystitis. Scand J Urol Nephrol 19:21–26.

Holm-Bentzen M, Jacobsen F, Nerstrom B et al. (1987a) Painful bladder disease: clinical and pathoanatomical differences in 115 patients. J Urol 138:500–502

Holm-Bentzen M, Søndergaard I, Hald T (1987b) Urinary excretion of a metabolite of histamine (1,4-methyl-imidazole-acetic-acid) in painful bladder disease. Br J Urol 59:230–233

Hunner GL (1915) A rare type of bladder ulcer in women: report of cases. Boston Med Surg J 172:660–664

Larsen S, Thompson SA, Hald T et al. (1982) Mast cells in interstitial cystitis. Br J Urol 54:283–286

Lose G, Frandsen B, Holm-Bentzen M, Larsen S, Jacobsen F (1987) Urine eosinophil cationic protein in painful bladder disease. Br J Urol 60:39–42

Lynes WL, Flynn SD, Shortliffe LD et al. (1987) Mast cell involvement in interstitial cystitis. J Urol 138:746–752

Meares Jr EMM (1987) Interstitial cystitis – 1987. Urology [Suppl] 29(4):46–48

Messing EM (1987) The diagnosis of interstitial cystitis. Urology [Suppl] 29(4):4–7

Messing EM, Stamey TA (1978) Interstitial cystitis. Early diagnosis, pathology and treatment. Urology 12:381–392

Oravisto KJ (1975) Epidemiology of interstitial cystitis. Ann Chir Gynaecol Fenn 64:75–77

Perez-Marrero R, Emerson L, Juma S (1987) Urodynamic studies in interstitial cystitis. Urology [Suppl] 29(4:27–30

Sant GR (1987) Intravesical 50% dimethyl sulfoxide (Rimso^5 – 50) in the treatment of interstitial cystitis. Urology [Suppl] 25(4):17–21

Simmons JL, Bunce PL (1958) On the use of an antihistamine in the treatment of interstitial cystitis. Am Surg 24:664–667

Smith BH, Dehner LP (1972) Chronic ulcerating cystitis. A study of 28 cases. Arch Pathol 93:76–81

Utz DC, Zincke H (1974) The masquerade of bladder cancer in situ as interstitial cystitis. J Urol 111:160–161

Webster GD, Galloway N (1987) Surgical treatment of interstitial cystitis: indications, techniques, and results. Urology [Suppl] 29(4):34–39

Chapter 11

Neurourologic Evaluation in Interstitial Cystitis

E. McGuire

Introduction

Uncomfortable urinary frequency is a common symptom, probably the most common symptom in urologic practice. Urologists would like urodynamic testing to provide information which helps to make a firm diagnosis in patients with this symptom; but unfortunately urodynamics cannot usually provide that. Without a great deal of additional background information, neurourologic techniques have little to offer as a first step in the investigation of patients with this kind of symptomatology.

Urgency and Frequency

These are subjective symptoms which can be roughly divided into two broad groups based on causality. *Sensory urgency* refers to the subjective sensation of the need to urinate and is almost never associated with urinary incontinence. The vast majority of patients with "interstitial cystitis" either the so-called early variety, or the more severe form of the disease, characterized by a physical limitation in vesical capacity, do not suffer from urinary incontinence. *Motor urgency* on the other hand is associated with urinary incontinence and presumably the uncomfortable urgency is related to an actual bladder contraction. Sensory urgency prompts frequent voiding to get rid of the symptom, which is usually not related to bladder volume as it is in normal individuals. This leads to the failure of frequent voiding to alleviate completely the symptom of urgency and to a frustrated patient. Motor urgency also often prompts frequent voiding but in this case the frequent voiding is a protective measure to avoid urinary incontinence. Since the symptoms are similar or nearly identical, it would seem logical to simply do a cystometrogram to determine whether the urgency is motor or sensory in character. Unfortunately, that does not work out very well in practice.

Cystometrograms and Other Urodynamic Tests and Uncomfortable Bladder Symptoms

Motor urgency is characterized by a detrusor contraction which occurs without its owners permission. This can result from various causes as spinal neural disease or obstructive uropathy, but may also be ideopathic. Bladder instability associated with neural disease or obstruction is relatively easily provoked by bladder filling and tends to occur at a smaller than normal bladder volume and is quite reproducible. Idiopathic instability as, for example, nocturnal eneuresis in children is not so easily characterized urodynamically. There is good evidence that idiopathic instability may be less a motor phenomenon than a sensory one. Patients with this problem show very poor appreciation of the degree of bladder filling and have an inadequate "early warning system" in that the first sensation of bladder activity is that associated with "urine passing" related to sudden unanticipated reflex vesical contractility. Detrusor instability associated with definite neural disease or obstructive uropathy responds predictably to anticholinergic agents (even if that response is not always equatable with continence (McGuire and Savastano 1983).

The idiopathic variety responds less predictably, and sometimes not at all. Whether the poor early warning system has a cortical, subcortical, or other basis is not clear at this time. Eneuretic children during sleep simply show no cortical arousal response to bladder filling to capacity in constrast to normal children (Kahn et al. 1984; Norgaard et al. 1984). Children with day and night-time incontinence will often demonstrate a reflex bladder contraction elicited by bladder filling which they cannot control and which occurs very suddenly. But this demonstration usually requires considerable distraction of the child from the circumstances of the urodynamic testing.

Adults are not so easily distracted, and the urodynamic test itself tends to obviate one of the problems in patients with ideopathic motor urge incontinence, which is poor cerebral appreciation of bladder filling. The results of several recent studies done in patients with urge incontinence by history suggest that continuous telemetric monitoring of bladder pressure while patients go about daily activities will often demonstrate bladder instability to be the cause of the patients' urge incontinence when a standard cystometrogram will not (Bradley et al. 1982; Thuroff et al. 1980).

While this chapter is not concerned with detrusor instability *per se*, these findings indicate that a cystometrogram is a relatively blunt instrument. The test misses approximately half of those with idiopathic detrusor instability. Moreover, a trial of anticholinergic agents based on a diagnosis made by history may not be successful simply because the abnormality is not related to true motor hyperactivity but rather to a poor warning and response system. What exists here is a normal reflex bladder response to filling which is a coordinated, facilitated reflex bladder contraction associated with urethral relaxation. As with most normal function, it responds poorly to medication designed to stop hyperreflexive activity. Of spinal cord injury patients with lesions superior to the sacral cord segments (upper motor neuron lesions) 85%–90% will respond to anticholinergic agents sufficiently well to become continent on a 4–6 hour intermittent catheterization schedule (McGuire and Savastano 1983). Giving 5 mg of Ditropan three times a day to the normal population would be unlikely to have the same result, nor are the results of treatment of patients with idiopathic instability very exciting. Neither are the results of treatment of patients with interstitial cystitis with anticholinergic agents good.

Urethral Activity and Uncomfortable Bladder Symptoms

Sudden, periodic, changes in urethral pressure have been associated by some workers with uncomfortable bladder symptoms as has urethral sphincter hyperactivity. Pronounced falls in urethral closing pressure measured in the urethral high pressure zone are chiefly the result of fluctuation in striated sphincter activity. Occasionally, a very pronounced fall in the urethral closing pressure, with opening of the vesical outlet which is normally closed by smooth muscle, can be observed urodynamically (McGuire 1978). This may be associated with urgency and urge incontinence. In these cases no bladder contractile activity or bladder contractility, which is of very low pressure, has been measured.

Urine entering the urethra can give rise to symptoms in some patients. However, at present, there are no substantive clinical or experimental findings which would permit urologists to use urethral pressure to make a definitive diagnosis of a condition which if treated would resolve uncomfortable bladder symptoms, i.e. urgency and frequency.

Urethral striated sphincter activity is associated with inhibition of detrusor contractility. Indeed, this is the single measurable effect when one asks a patient who is voiding to stop. Experimentally and clinically, stimulation of the external urethral sphincter, pelvic floor, or perineal nerve or the sacral nerve roots can result in inhibition of reflex detrusor contractility (Glenn 1973; McGuire et al. 1983). Hyperactivity of this area in patients with bladder instability or uncomfortable bladder symptoms is not a surprising finding. Neither is it surprising that external sphincter activity varies during bladder filling, particularly in the circumstances of urodynamic testing. On the other hand, internal sphincter activity is clearly related in a direct way to reflex detrusor contractility in that maintenance of urethral closure at the bladder neck is normally interrupted only by reflex bladder contractility. Thus, contrary to much of the earlier literature, opening of the internal sphincter is a neural event, driven by the same parasympathetic discharge which excites a bladder contraction. At the present time, we have not defined precisely what activity in the urethra is abnormal, nor have we linked some particular pattern of activity to a disease or even a symptom complex in a definitive way. One could not make a diagnosis from an isolated urodynamic tracing, however sophisticated, if one knew nothing about the patient. It is quite likely that we will be able to catagorize various types of somatic and smooth sphincter activity, normal and abnormal. But at present, we cannot do that as we can in other conditions. Obstructive uropathy, for example, can be measured best by the effect of that process on bladder pressure at the time of micturition. A urethra which functions poorly on radiographic evaluation can be related to symptomatic involuntary urinary loss. These relatively familiar and straightforward relationships are not quite the same as the "urethral syndrome" or "disorders of urethral compliance" or "sphincter hyperactivity" about which we know very little, particularly the relationship of the observed changes to symptoms.

Assessment of Bladder Compliance (Ability to Tolerate Volume Increments) and Interstitial Cystitis

There are two basic abnormalities in patients with interstitial cystitis, one of which is entirely subjective in character. The patient's report of the volume required to initiate urgency, which may be intense, is nevertheless subjective. In most patients with interstitial cystitis, subjective discomfort is provoked at smaller volumes than normal despite the fact that the bladder will physically tolerate larger volumes easily. It is not clear what generates this uncomfortable response. Incremental volume clearly makes it worse, but volume alone or stretch and tension may not be primarily involved as usually very small volumes are required to initiate discomfort. Neither is it clear that the painful sensation is in every instance carried via sensory fibers traveling with the pelvic nerves. These fibers enter the sacral cord via the sacral roots, the same sacral roots which subserve reflex bladder function. That kind of neural activity, if intense enough, might be expected to generate, with the pain, a reflex bladder response which does not occur.

There is an interesting group of patients collected by most urodynamic centers over time whose difficulties begin with gross prolonged overdistension of the bladder, which when corrected by catheter drainage or intermittent catheterization gradually leads to totally uninhibitable reflex bladder contractility with absolutely no bladder sensation at all. Such patients do not respond to anticholinergic agents and often end up with a urinary diversion. These patients do, however, provide clinical information which suggests that sensory information which excites vesical contractility is not the same as that which provokes the sensation of urgency. Urgency may be conveyed by afferent fibers other than those which subserve reflex bladder activity. Because bladder inflammation resulting from bacterial infection can cause identical symptoms, we have not unreasonably assumed that inflammation may be the etiology of the uncomfortable symptoms in patients with interstitial cystitis. However, there is no real proof for that concept, and the actual cause of the uncomfortable bladder symptoms in interstitial cystitis remains unknown, as does the tissue receptor or tissue site which is responsible for the generation of the symptoms. Neither is the neural pathway which conveys the sensation of discomfort clearly known.

Urodynamic Testing and Physical Volume Restriction

Some patients with interstitial cystitis tolerate bladder filling poorly and manifest on cystometric testing, awake or when fully anesthetized, a rise in bladder pressure with increasing volume which at some point simply shuts off the infusion. This kind of poorly compliant bladder is associated with overt endoscopic findings including gross bleeding, ulceration, edema and trabeculation. This kind of badly damaged bladder does not respond to more conservative measures of treatment and usually requires partial cystectomy and augmentation cystoplasty. Results in such patients are usually excellent with immediate relief of pain. Such patients easily accept the necessity of intermittent catherization and a long difficult procedure very readily. The chief differential diagnoses in these patients are carcinoma in situ, radiation cystitis, and very occasionally a poorly inhibited bladder or a decentralized bladder. The surgical procedure is basically designed to achieve low pressure reservoir capability.

Patients with uncomfortable symptoms but with normal bladder capacities under anesthesia are a different problem. Operative results are not generally good in such patients and bladder augmentation and partial cystectomy is often followed by cystectomy and urinary diversion. There is little or no evidence that this variety of what we have chosen to call interstitial cystitis progresses to the more virulent clinical variety described above. Indeed, the mechanism of the diseases may be entirely different. The true natural history of the disease in these patients as opposed to those with progressive difficulty remains unknown. Urodynamic studies may suggest improvement or worsening of the symptoms when related to bladder volume, but these studies really do not help with assessment of response to treatment since in many such patients the disease waxes and wanes in an untreated state. Moreover, there is very little evidence that treatment does anything more than influence the symptomatic expression of the disease rather than cure the condition which may occur spontaneously.

References

Bradley WE, Bhatia N, Haldeman S (1982) 24-hour continuous monitoring. Proc Am Urol Assoc 113:497 (abstract)

Glenn E (1973) Control of incontinence by electrical devises. In: Caldwell KPS (ed) Urinary incontinence. Grune and Stratton, New York (1983) pp 89–109

Kahn Z, Meiza M, Leiter E (1984) Role of detrusor hyperreflexia (bladder instability) in primary eneuresis. Proceedings of the International Continence Society, Innsbruck, 1984, pp 107–108

McGuire EJ (1978) Reflex urethral instability. Br J Urol 50:200–204

McGuire EJ, Savastano JA (1983) Long-term follow-up of spinal cord injury patients managed by intermittent catheterization. J Urol 129:775–778

McGuire EJ, Shin-Chun Z, Horwinski ER, Lytton B (1983) Treatment of motor and sensory instability by electrical stimulation. J Urol 129:78–79

Norgaard JP, Knudsen N, Hansen JH, Neilson JB, Djurhuus JC (1984) Overnight monitoring of children with nocturnal eneuresis. Proceedings of the International Continence Society, Innsbruck, 1984, pp 105–106

Thuroff JW, Jonas U, Froneberg D et al. (1980) Telemetric urodynamic investigations in normal males. Urol Int 35:427–430

Chapter 12

Hydrodistension and Intraoperative Urodynamics

A. Nehra and Y. Vardi

Introduction

Hydrodistension of the bladder has served as both a diagnostic modality and as one of the mainstays of therapy in patients suspected of and diagnosed with interstitial cystitis (Hanno and Wein 1987). Since Hunner (1915) first recommended local excision of the "elusive ulcer" numerous therapeutic modalities, among them intravesical hydrodistension often in combination with intravesical instillation (see Chap. 14) has been recommended.

History of Intravesical Hydrodistension

Distension of the bladder by hydraulic distension (Bumpus 1930), balloon catheter (Kearns 1932), tidal irrigation (Longacre 1936), delayed micturition (Ormond 1937), and condom balloon (Bohne and Fetz 1954) have been utilized in the treatment of interstitial cystitis (Messing and Stamey 1978).

The technique of hydrodistension of the bladder was popularized as a therapeutic modality by Karl Helmstein for the treatment of carcinoma of the urinary bladder. Helmstein described two techniques of hydrodistension, the objective of both being to maintain the intravesical pressure close to the patient's diastolic blood pressure for a duration of 5–6 hours in order to induce tumor necrosis. Distension was achieved with a Foley catheter alone, or with an intravesical balloon (Helmstein 1966, 1972).

Helmstein's Technique

Saline Infusion With Foley Catheter

A 70 cm water pressure was obtained by adjusting the height of the infusion set. Saline was infused through a Foley catheter and approximately 1000 ml was usually required to attain the required pressure in patients with carcinoma of the urinary bladder. Escape of the fluid was prevented by pulling the balloon of the catheter against the bladder neck.

Intravesical Placement of a Rubber Balloon

A 16 Fr Foley catheter was completely divided at its tip, and a steel tube which was used as a stent was threaded through the Foley. An internal steel sleeve was placed at the tip of the Foley in order to provide reinforcement. A distensible rubber balloon was drawn over and fastened behind the Foley catheter's own balloon. The stent was then advanced in order to extend the balloon so that it could be passed through a resectoscope. The resectoscope was withdrawn after inflating the Foley balloon and saline infusion was started at 20 ml increments to a pressure of 100 cm H_2O (recognizing that a 25 cm water pressure was required to overcome the additional elasticity of the balloon).

Utilizing Helmstein's technique of hydrodistension (except to a pressure equivalent to the patients systolic blood pressure), Dunn (1974) initially treated 20 patients with bladder instability and subsequently (1977) used prolonged hydrodistension in 25 patients with a diagnosis of interstitial cystitis. Of 25 patients 16 were symptom free and demonstrated an increased bladder capacity (approximately three times the pretreatment capacity) at a mean duration of 14 months.

The mechanism of action of bladder hydrodistension is at present unknown. It is postulated that hydrodistension may result in ischemia or physical damage to the mucosa, nervous tissue or muscle wall of the urinary bladder. Since the mucosa and submucosa are subjected to the maximal effect of bladder hydrodistension, damage to the submucosal afferent nerve plexus may be responsible for improvement of symptoms. Experimental work performed on animal models by Sehn (1976) demonstrated axonal degeneration to occur immediately following hydrodistension of the bladder, however it is not known whether normal function resumes following regeneration of the axons.

Hydrodistension of the bladder is generally the initial therapeutic modality used in the treatment of patients with interstitial cystitis, and may be performed at the time of the initial cystoscopic procedure. Messing (1986) as well as Hanno and Wein (1987) reported symptomatic improvement in 30% of the patients following the procedure.

While currently there is no standard regimen used for hydrodistension as a therapeutic modality, we distend the bladder, using irrigation fluid to a peak intravesical pressure of 80 cm H_2O (utilizing cystometric monitoring) for a duration of 8–10 minutes. At the termination of the procedure, after the bladder is emptied, a solution consisting of one ampoule of bicarbonate, 5 000 units heparin, 10 mg Kenalog and 50 mg 50% DMSO in 50 ml is instilled in the bladder and the catheter clamped until the patient is uncomfortable in the recovery room. The bladder is then emptied and the catheter withdrawn.

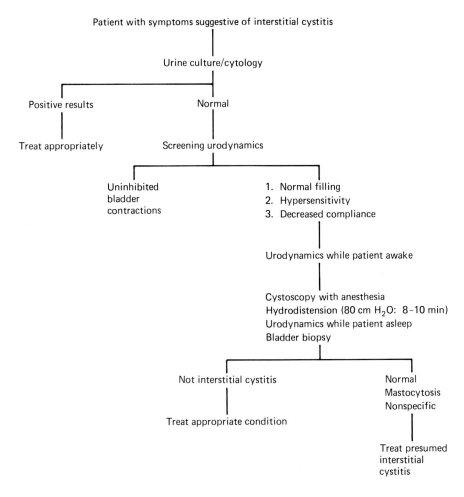

Fig. 12.1. Diagnosis: the evaluation of patients.

Diagnosis

The increased incidence of diagnosis of interstitial cystitis may be attributed to increased awareness by urologists. Conversely, the commonest reason for the diagnosis to be missed is a failure to consider interstitial cystitis during the evaluation of chronic lower urinary tract symptomatology.

The evaluation of patients requires a systematic approach (Fig.12.1). Endoscopy and bladder biopsy (to rule out other pathology) under anesthesia in conjunction with hydrodistension of the bladder are important in establishing the presumptive diagnosis of interstitial cystitis.

The use of hydrodistension as a diagnostic modality was established by Messing and Stamey (1978). They described the presence of pin-point petechial hemorrhages, occasionally seen during the first filling of the bladder, but appearing throughout the vesical submucosa on second hydrodistension of the bladder. These "glomerulations" (red strawberry-like dots) coalesce to become hemorrhagic spots which ooze blood. Glomerulations are seen mostly on the dome and posterior wall of the bladder and are thought to represent the hallmark of the diagnosis of interstitial cystitis, although they are not pathognomonic of the condition.

Complications

Complications following hydrodistension of the bladder (Ramsden et al. 1976; Higson et al. 1978) include bladder rupture, hematuria, backache, and urinary retention.

The incidence of bladder rupture during prolonged distension of 113 patients with a diagnosis of detrusor instability, interstitial cystitis, reduced bladder capacity of unknown etiology and post-irradiation bladder fibrosis was 8%. Experience from this series suggested that bladder wall disease may be an important factor in the pathogenesis of bladder rupture. The site of rupture was usually at the vault or at the junction of the posterior and superior walls of the bladder. Following intraperitoneal or extraperitoneal rupture conservative management (catheter drainage) was performed, with complete bladder healing in all patients. Rupture of the bladder did not adversely affect the outcome of prolonged distension, and the quality of improvement in some of these patients appeared to be enhanced. Hematuria, backache, and retention are present for a short duration and patients were usually asymptomatic in a few days.

Intraoperative Urodynamics During Hydrodistension

In addition to bladder hydrodistension, we currently use intraoperative cystometry to provide more accurate information about bladder compliance during our diagnostic evaluation. Cystometry may be performed simultaneously with the cystoscopic evaluation and hydrodistension therapy through the outflow port of a continuous flow resectoscope (or following a screening cystoscopy through a continuous flow Foley).

The intitial filling is performed with the patient awake at a fast (125 ml/min) filling rate. The volume and the intravesical pressure at which the first sensation, feeling of fullness, mild pain, and severe pain (maximal bladder capacity) are noted. Anesthesia is induced, and the distension is repeated with continuous monitoring of the intravesical volume and pressure. An intravesical pressure of 80 cm H_2O is maintained for 8–10 minutes. Additional volume is often required to maintain this pressure due to delayed bladder accommodation.

Perez-Marrero et al. (1987) reported their urodynamic findings in patients diagnosed as having interstitial cystitis. These were: frequency, urgency, suprapubic discomfort relieved by voiding, the cystoscopic finding of bladder glomerulation after distension, and the histologic finding of mast cells in the

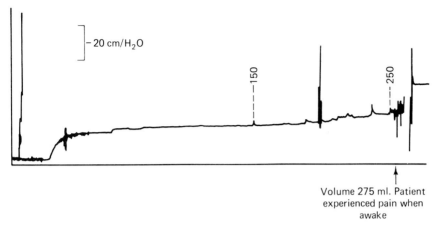

Fig. 12.2. Slow fill cystometry (50 ml/min) performed with the patient awake. Total volume infused is 275 ml, when patient experienced severe pain. Increase in intravesical pressure is 10 cm H_2O above baseline.

biopsies obtained of the bladder muscularis. All 50 patients had normal uroflowmetry and residual urine, and none exhibited detrusor sphincter dyssynergia. On cystometric examination (while awake) all showed bladder hypersensitivity (first sensation of filling: 100 ml), and no decrease in compliance was noted. Uninhibited bladder contractions were noted in 26% of the patients. The maximum cystometric capacity was 50–615 ml (mean 287 ml). A trend toward smaller bladder capacities was noted in patients with a longer duration of symptoms.

Our urodynamic findings (unpublished) in 20 patients with interstitial cystitis differ somewhat from these observations. A normal uroflow, minimal post-void residual, and coordinated bladder and sphincter function were found to be consistent with the prior report. However, in our 20 cases we did not have any patient with bladder instability. The maximal cystometric capacities (awake) varied from 45 ml to 350 ml (mean 275 ml).

Cystometry following the induction of anaesthesia allowed bladder filling beyond the pain tolerance of the patient, and provided an objective assessment

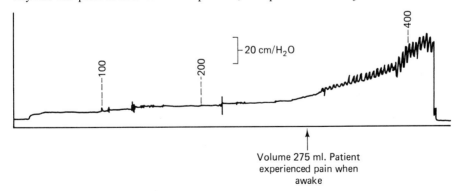

Fig. 12.3. Slow fill cystometry (50 ml/min) performed with patient under general anesthesia. Total volume infused is 420 ml. Non-compliance (50 cm H_2O pressure rise per 100 ml infused) begins at approximately 300 ml bladder volume.

of bladder compliance (Figs 12.2, 12.3). We have observed a relationship among the values for voided volumes (daily diary and voided volume charts), cystometric volume at first sensation (slow and fast fill cystometry), maximal cystometric capacity (fast fill capacity at which severe discomfort is noted), and the volume at which significant non-compliance is noted (greater than 15 cm H_2O pressure rise per 50 ml of fluid infused at 125 ml/min while under anesthesia.

The voided volumes (determined from the patient's bladder diaries) usually approximated the first sensation at bladder filling during cystometry. The onset of severe pain during cystometry, approximated twice the typical voided volume (Fig 12.2). Only 20% of the patients were able to tolerate an intravesical pressure greater than 20 cm H_2O above the baseline while awake. Three of these four patients were able to tolerate fast fill cystometry (125 ml/min) while awake to a pressure 30 cm H_2O above the baseline. Under anesthesia, 16 of the 20 patients demonstrated non-compliance (elevation of intravesical pressure greater than 15 cm H_2O for 50 ml volume) within 100 ml of the volume at which they noted severe pain when awake (Figs 12.3, 12.4, 12.5). Maximal cystometric capacity (volume required to generate and maintain an intravesical pressure of 80 cm H_2O) while anesthetized averaged 674 ml ($\pm$ 232 ml). Spinal anesthesia in 3 patients did not effect the demonstration of non-compliance. The addition of intravenous atropine (0.01 mg/kg) prior to the induction of anesthesia did not affect the cystometric parameters while awake (performed in the first 8 patients only).

These results suggest an association between the volume associated with the onset of severe pain and the development of non-compliance (Figs. 12.3, 12.4, 12.5). A cause and effect relationship – does frequent voiding accentuate non-compliance, or does the development of non-compliance decrease the volume which can be tolerated until severe pain is experienced – cannot be

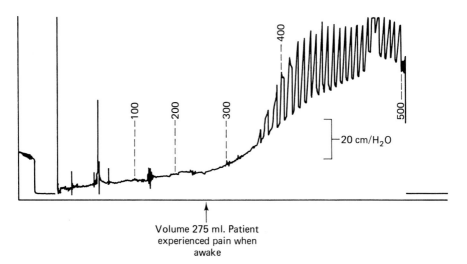

Volume 275 ml. Patient
experienced pain when
awake

Fig. 12.4. Fast fill cystometry (125 ml/min) performed with the patient under general anesthesia. Non-compliance is again demonstrated at approximtely 300 ml bladder volume. (Increases in intra-abdominal pressure from ventilation are evident).

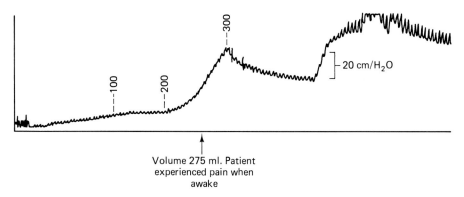

300

100

200

20 cm/H$_2$O

↑
Volume 275 ml. Patient
experienced pain when
awake

Fig. 12.5. Fast fill cystometry (125 ml/min) performed with the patient under general anesthesia. The infusion is stopped at 300 ml and bladder accommodation is noted. Non-compliance is again demonstrated when the infusion is restarted.

established. A physical change in the bladder wall, as opposed to a neurologic mechanism may be implied by the persistence of non-compliance by the use of spinal anesthetic.

Conclusion

Although hydrodistension was first introduced as a therapeutic modality, it is at present one of the mainstays in diagnosing patients with interstitial cystitis. Therapeutic hydrodistension and intravesical therapy has been demonstrated to be a relatively safe and easily performed procedure, which can be performed at the time of diagnostic hydrodistension. A variable symptomatic response of approximately 30% has been reported by several investigators.

Intraoperative cystometry can be performed in conjunction with hydrodistension for accurate monitoring of the intravesical pressure and noncompliance. The usefulness of the information obtained by objective measurement of decreased bladder compliance under anesthesia to the diagnosis and therapy of interstitial cystitis should be further investigated, since it may provide an additional criterion for classifying patients and their response to therapy.

References

Bohne AW, Fetz RJ (1954) Interstitial cystitis: an adjunct in its treatment. Arch Surg 69:831–837
Bumpus HC (1930) Interstitial cystitis: its treatment by overdistension of the bladder. Med Clin North Am 13:1495–1499
Dunn M, Smith JC, Ardran, GM (1974) Prolonged bladder distension as a treatment of urgency and urge incontinence of urine. Br J Urol 46:645–652
Dunn M, Ramsden PD, Roberts JBM, Smith JC, Smith PJB (1977) Interstitial cystitis, treated by prolonged bladder distension. Br J Urol 49:641–645.

Hanno PM, Wein AJ (1987) Interstitial cystitis, part II. AUA update series, lesson 10, vol VI.

Helmstein K (1966) Hydrostatis pressure therapy. A new approach to the treatment of carcinoma of the bladder. Opuscula Medica (Stockh) 9:238–243

Helmstein K (1972) Treatment of bladder carcinoma by a hydrostatic pressure technique. Br J Urol 44:434–450

Higson RH, Smith JC, Whelan P (1978) Bladder rupture: an acceptable complication of distension therapy. Br J Urol 50:529–534

Hunner GL (1915) A rare type of bladder ulcer in women; report of cases. Boston Med Surg J 172:660–664

Kearns WM (1932) A new method to bring about dilatation of the contracted bladder. Urol Cut Rev 36:184–186.

Longacre JJ (1936) The treatment of contracted bladder with controlled tidal irrigation. J Urol 36:25–31.

Messing EM (1986) Interstitial cystitis and related syndromes. In: Walsh PC et al. (eds) Campbell's urology, 4th edn. Saunders, Philadelphia, pp 1070–1092

Messing EM, Stamey TA (1978) Interstitial cystitis: early diagnosis, pathology and treatment. Urology 12:381–392

Ormond JK (1937) Interstitial cystitis. J Urol 33:376–380

Perez-Marrero R, Emerson L, Juma S (1987) Urodynamic studies in interstitial cystitis. Urology [suppl] 29:27–32

Ramsden PD, Smith JC, Dunn M, Ardraw, GM (1976) Distension therapy for the unstable bladder: later results including an assessment of repeat distensions. Br J Urol 48:623–629

Sehn JT (1976) The ultrastructural effect of prolonged distension on the neuromuscular apparatus of the bladder. MSc thesis, University of Oxford.

Editorial Comment

The Clinical Evaluation of Patients with Painful Bladder Disease

A.R. Stone

We believe the most important factor in the diagnosis of interstitial cystitis is a heightened index of suspicion. The majority of patients in our series have seen, on average, three physicians, often including urologists and gynecologists, before the diagnosis of interstitial cystitis is even entertained. It is astounding to find so many patients given the diagnosis of recurrent urinary tract infection, and treated with multiple courses of antibiotics, without positive urine cultures.

A significant proportion of our patients are referred to the urodynamics laboratory because of frequency and urgency. Careful attention to history in these patients will identify the common component of suprapubic pain. Urodynamically, patients are invariably stable and void efficiently, but exhibit detrusor hypersensitivity with early first sensation of filling and a low cystometric capacity. Contrary to previously held beliefs, compliance is almost always normal, as the patient will not allow bladder filling to an extent where impaired compliance may be elicited.

Some patients will describe fairly bizarre symptoms. I believe these are due partly to varying perceptions of this visceral pain, and in part to the anxiety engendered by the absence of a reasonable diagnosis. I recently evaluated a patient who I was convinced had a bladder pheochromocytoma, experiencing severe palpitations during and after voiding. This condition was excluded and the diagnosis of interstitial cystitis was confirmed endoscopically and pathologically.

Although the diagnosis should be confirmed by endoscopy and biopsy, we believe the histological criteria are still not specific enough. Before committing patients to cystoscopy, we usually instruct them to keep a voiding chart and, if possible, try and increase the time interval between voids. This allows the physician to obtain an objective assessment of their voiding behavior and will potentially allow a percentage of patients with less severe forms of bladder hypersensitivity to improve clinically and thus not require further intervention. This conservative form of assessment may also allow the identification of those patients who may benefit from other forms of behavioral therapy or neurostimulation techniques.

If no improvement is experienced on bladder training, we agree with the need for cystoscopy under general anesthetic to confirm the diagnosis. We have routinely carried this out under a light general anesthetic in order to determine the bladder volume at which a sensory response is obtained. The anesthesiologist monitors respiratory and heart rates, and notes the volume at which these rise, giving a further parameter in the assessment of disease severity. We distend the bladder for one minute with the irrigating fluid at 80–100 cm H_2O above the bladder, and repeat this if no glomerulations are seen after this first distension.

Following this, several biopsies are taken using cold cup forceps. If carried out correctly, this technique can provide adequate sampling of both submucosa and muscularis. A recent survey of our last 25 biopsies, taken in this way for interstitial cystitis, failed to obtain muscle in only two cases. We also take biopsies from the trigone to evaluate the extent of disease.

Fulguration and postoperative catheter drainage are very important as these patients have a propensity to hemorrhage. The catheter can usually be removed the following morning.

It is important to specifically ask the pathologist to stain for mast cells (Giemsa's or toluidine blue stain) as well as H&E. Trichrome stain is also helpful in assessing the amount of fibrous tissue in the biopsy. Without this pathological direction, a diagnosis of chronic cystitis only is the usual answer received.

It is rare to find patients with the so-called classic form of the disease, contracted bladder, or Hunner's ulcer, but it is agreed that these patients will not respond to conservative therapy. The majority of patients seen in our series are the so-called early form, with normal mucosa initially, and glomerulations or petechiae following hydrodistension.

The extent of glomerulations and capacity under general anesthetic bear little relationship to the severity of symptoms and, thus, we will only use these findings to confirm the diagnosis and not to absolutely dictate therapy although there is some evidence that patients with large capacities under anesthetic do not respond well to any form of surgical reconstruction.

In order to make the diagnosis of interstitial cystitis, typical endoscopic findings need not always be present. If the symptoms are typical and biopsy shows a chronic inflammatory infiltrate with any degree of mastocytosis in either muscularis or submucosa or both, we will accept these criteria as being confirmatory of interstitial cystitis. Whether in time, with more accurate diagnostic criteria, we will be able to differentiate various types of painful bladder disease in this population remains to be seen.

Other diagnostic modalities such as measurement of eosinophilic cationic protein may provide more simple and effective methods of evaluating these patients.

The use of flow cytometry in this disease is controversial. Interstitial cystitis is generally a disease of the submucosa and muscularis, and most patients will have normal appearing epithelium despite severe disease in deeper layers. Flow cytometry measures DNA content in cells shed in the urine, presumably epithelial cells. Thus, it is expecting a lot of this technique to be able to discern abnormalities in cells probably not involved in the disease process. Our experience with this modality is similar to that of the authors, with normal results obtained in every case.

Finally, once the diagnosis is confirmed, it is important to explain the nature of the condition to the patient. A definite diagnosis, and a sympathetic physician, will help to alleviate much anxiety. This interview and subsequent interviews during initial treatment are important in the overall clinical evaluation of the patient with interstitial cystitis. If conservative measures do not work and surgical intervention is contemplated, this partly psychologic evaluation may be extremely helpful in deciding the appropriateness of reconstructive procedures or urinary diversion.

Interstitial Cystitis

G.S. Benson

John Hunner's "elusive" ulcer has eluded me. I see many patients who "should" have a Hunner's ulcer, but I have yet to find one. I see many patients who "should" have interstitial cystitis, but I am not sure I can define the disease, let alone diagnose it. I am hesitant to tell my patients that they have "painful bladder disease". They already know they have bladder pain, and I have very little, either diagnostically or therapeutically, to add.

"Painful bladder disease", I think, clinically defines itself. A definition, either clinical or pathological, of interstitial cystitis is desperately needed. Although such findings as increased numbers of mast cells in the detrusor muscle may prove in the future to define interstitial cystitis, at present the pathologic findings are nonspecific and clinicians are forced to accept a clinical definition.

The clinical diagnosis of "interstitial cystitis" includes the presence of frequency, dysuria, and pain in the absence of identifiable cause. The hallmark of the clinical diagnosis is, I think, the presence of mucosal hemorrhage or "glomerulations" seen at cystoscopy. These changes are also, however, nonspecific, and may in fact be seen in patients who have no symptoms whatsoever. I biopsy many of these patients, not to make the diagnosis of interstitial cystitis (because I do not know what to look for), but to rule out the presence of carcinoma in situ (CIS). CIS may masquerade as "interstitial cystitis", but no existing data support the concept that "interstitial cystitis" (whatever the definition) is a premalignant lesion.

Many patients have debilitating bladder symptoms. A few present with very small bladder capacities and such severe symptoms that operative therapy is warranted. Most patients, however, present with symptoms and very few, if any, objective findings. Although meaningful research is currently underway, we must be careful not to pretend to understand a symptom complex we cannot with accuracy clinically (let alone pathologically) define.

We may be doing our patients a disservice by diagnosing "interstitial cystitis". I would much prefer to say "I believe you have symptoms, I don't know what's wrong with you, but I'll do my best to make you symptomatically better". Patients now, however, generally demand more. Nevertheless, we should not be so enthralled by the current publicity surrounding "interstitial cystitis" that we are afraid to say "I don't know".

Section 4
Management

Chapter 13

Pharmacotherapeutic Goals in Interstitial Cystitis

K.-E. Andersson and H. Hedlund

The classic symptoms of interstitial cystitis include unremitting frequency, urgency and suprapubic or pelvic pain (Messing 1986; Parivar and Bradbrook 1986) Irrespective of what is causing these symptoms the most urgent pharmacotherapeutic goal should be to make the patient symptom-free. However, this goal seems difficult to achieve and most textbooks and reviews stress that treatment is unsatisfactory both from a clinical and scientific point of view (Messing 1986; Parivar and Bradbrook 1986). With available modalities, the majority of patients can obtain relief of symptoms, but rarely will these be totally or permanently eliminated (Messing 1986; Hanno and Wein 1987).

The ultimate goal of pharmacotherapy is of course to neutralize the factor(s) causing the disease. However, as long as causative factors are unknown, treatments will be based on empiricism. It cannot be excluded that a positive response to drugs with known mechanisms of action may give some information on the factors causing the disease. So far, this line of research has borne little fruit. It should, however, continue to be a goal of future pharmacotherapy to contribute to the elucidation of the etiology and pathogenesis of the disorder.

The list of drugs which have been used for treatment of interstitial cystitis is long and extremely variable (see, e.g., Messing 1986). This may reflect not only the uncertainty of the etiology of the disease, but also that the methods for evaluation of therapeutic interventions have been inadequate. Even if restricted to what can be regarded as currently used therapy the drug list is long (Table 13.1).

When reviewing the documentation for the efficacy of different treatments, the absence of controlled clinical trials is striking. This may have several explanations, but nevertheless makes it difficult to assess drug efficacy. Much of the documentation is old and does not meet with the modern requirements of clinical trials. Patient materials are sometimes small and/or inhomogenous and criteria for diagnosis and effect evaluation not well defined. It is obvious that most of the "accepted" therapy today is based more on clinical impressions than on controlled clinical trials. As stated by Wein (1985) "drawing conclusions about etiology or treatment from results obtained with non-randomized 'built-up' therapy without controls can be totally misleading". There is always a

Table 13.1. Current drug
treatment of interstitial cystitis

Systemic treatment
  Corticosteroids
  Immunosuppressive drugs
  Anti-inflammatory drugs
  Antihistamines
  Pentosanpolyphosphate
  Heparin
  Amitriptyline

Local treatment
  Dimethyl sulfoxide (DMSO)
  Oxychlorosene sodium
    (Chlorpactin WCS 90)
  Silver nitrate
  Disodium chromoglycate

price to pay in terms of risks connected to effective drug therapy. Messing (1986) stressed that the disease offers little actual risk to health and life and that it is almost never a manifestation of an underlying disease that does present such a risk. It is therefore questionable whether a drug treatment with known serious adverse effects should be used, particularly if its efficacy has not been demonstrated in an acceptable way. An important immediate goal in pharmacotherapy is therefore to document the efficacy of current therapy in an acceptable way. A long list of "potentially" effective drugs serves neither the doctor nor the patient.

It is obvious that to be able to design good clinical trials several pieces of information about the course of the disease are needed. Thus it is desirable to establish the rate of spontaneous remissions. This would also make it possible, to some extent, to assess the effect of drug interventions as studied in open trials. Oravisto and Alfthan (1976) calculated, based on experience of 151 patients, a remission rate (remission lasting for at least 6 months) of 11% in patients with all grades of severity of the disease.

Due consideration must be given to some important factors. One is that strict diagnostic criteria are applied. Some of the reported differences in therapeutic efficacy may be due to differences in diagnostic criteria with resulting differences in patient material. Fall et al. (1987) suggested that ulcerative and non-ulcerative interstitial cystitis may be separate entities and also that the conditions should be evaluated separately in clinical studies.

A definition of what is a satisfactory response to treatment is desired. The ambitions seem to vary and what is called an excellent result by one investigator may be considered a poor response by another (De Juana and Everett 1977). If the therapy suppresses symptoms, but does not influence the disease process, it is essential that this is clarified. Symptom relief is not necessarily linked to morphological improvement.

The placebo response to treatment has to be estimated. In two controlled studies, one on the effects of oral pentosanpolysulfate (Holm-Bentzen et al. 1986b; 1987) and the other on intravesical DMSO (Perez-Marrero et al. 1986) the placebo response was high, up to 50%.

The efficacy and risks of different drug treatments should be evaluated, but pharmacotherapy should also be compared with other forms of nonsurgical treatment, e.g. hydrodistension (Dunn et al. 1977) and electrical nerve stimulation (Fall 1987). Combination of treatments may be effective.

As mentioned previously one of the immediate goals of pharmacotherapy of interstitial cystitis should be to document the efficacy of current treatments. This chapter reviews the list of "accepted" drug treatments of interstitial cystitis with the following questions in mind: What is the rationale for treatment? What is the basis for accepting a drug therapy as effective and what is the documented efficacy?

Corticosteroids

It is well documented that an inflammatory reaction of bladder structures is a characteristic of interstitial cystitis; histopathologically there is a generalized pancystitis (Fall et al. 1985; Holm-Bentzen and Lose 1987). It is therefore reasonable to expect a positive response to corticosteroids. Early studies on the effects of corticosteroids given orally or infiltrated into the bladder reported diverging results, but suggested that beneficial effects could be obtained in some patients (e.g. Hoyt 1952; Dees 1953; Johnston 1956; Franksson 1957; Kinder and Smith 1958; Guerrier et al. 1965).

In 1971 Badenoch reported his own therapeutic results in 56 cases of interstitial cystitis; of these, 25 were treated with systemic corticosteroids in a non-controlled way. After dilatation of the bladder, patients were treated with 15 mg prednisolone daily for a week, 10 mg daily for a week and then 5 mg daily for many months. No details were given but on this regimen 19 out of 25 cases were reported to have "sustained improvement" and were able to lead a "fairly normal life". Even if some patients were found to develop osteoporosis and fluid retention, Badenoch (1971) felt convinced that patients with chronic interstitial cystitis should always have an extensive trial on this therapy. This view was not shared by Walsh (1978) who considered the response to corticosteroids to be totally unpredictable and the dose needed to get a positive response considerable.

No controlled clinical trials seem to have been performed documenting the efficacy of systemically (or locally) given corticosteroids and clarifying the relation between efficacy and risks with long-term treatment. Such studies are to be desired.

Immunosuppressive Drugs

The basis for including immunosuppressive drugs among those used for current treatment of interstitial cystitis seems to be the report of Oravisto and Alfthan from 1976. Assuming the disease to be related to the autoimmune collagen diseases (Oravisto and Alfthan 1976; Oravisto et al. 1970) they gave azathioprine (initial dose 150 mg daily, maintenance dose 50–100 mg daily) to 38 patients and found pain to disappear completely in 22 and pollakiuria in 20 of them. Chloroquine or oxychloroquine usually combined with salicylate was tried in 22 patients and in 11 pain disappeared. Only 4 noted improvement in frequency. Ten patients in the azathioprine group and 8 patients in the chloroquine group did not respond. The improvement on azathioprine was noted in 1–2 weeks, but was very slow during chloroquine treatment, requiring up to 4–6 months. Side effects were not reported, nor were follow-up times.

There are no controlled clinical trials on the effects of immunosuppressive drugs in interstitial cystitis. Published experiences cannot be regarded as sufficient to assess their value in the treatment of this disorder.

Anti-Inflammatory Drugs

There are several anecdotal reports on the use of different anti-inflammatory drugs in the treatment of interstitial cystitis (e.g. Guerrier et al. 1965). Benzydamine (1-benzyl-3-[3(dimethylamino)propoxy]-1H-indazole) is one of these drugs. Like other non-steroid anti-inflammatory drugs, benzydamine inhibits cyclo-oxygenase, although its mode of action may not be identical with that of indomethacin or phenylbutazone (Gryglewski 1979; Shen 1979). It has not gained any wide use in treatment of patients with inflammatory disorders and it is not registered for systemic use in, for example, the Scandinavian countries.

Walsh (1977a) reported the results of an open study where 25 patients with interstitial cystitis were treated with 100 mg oral benzydamine twice daily. Pain, which was a predominant symptom was dramatically relieved in 18 patients, whereas frequency of micturition was improved to varying extent. Within 2–10 days of not taking the drug, pain recurred in most patients. Follow-up was 2 years. Walsh (1977b) later reported that a double-blind trial of benzydamine in interstitial cystitis was abandoned, because after 12 patients entering the trial no one had experienced any significant symptom relief.

On the basis of available information, it must be concluded that the efficacy of benzydamin and other non-steroid anti-inflammatory drugs remains unproven in interstitial cystitis.

Antihistamines

Several authors have suggested that mast cells may have a direct relation to the pathogenesis of interstitial cystitis and may also be used as a pathognomonic marker of the disease (see, e.g., Larsen et al. 1982; Holm-Bentzen and Lose 1987; Fall et al. 1987). It is well known that mast cells produce, among other compounds, histamine, and that histamine release in tissues may cause pain, hyperemia and fibrosis, all features which may characterize interstitial cystitis. Furthermore, Kastrup et al. (1983) found the histamine content of the bladder wall of interstitial cystitis patients to be increased.

There may thus be a rationale for the use of antihistimines in the treatment of interstitial cystitis, and these drugs are frequently included in the drug treatment of the disorder. However, the basis for accepting antihistamines as effective drug treatment is surprisingly weak. Simmons and Bunce (1958) reported three cases of interstitial cystitis responding to tripelennamine (Pyribenzamine, PBZ). The response was described as dramatic but two of the patients were treated with bladder dilation and silver nitrate instillations immediately before antihistamine treatment was started. Simmons (1961) reported on 6 cases responding positively to tripelennamine 50 mg 3 times daily. However, the response was not convincing in all patients and the duration of effect was quite variable. Cystoscopy showed no change of the appearance of the bladder, even when the response was satisfactory.

No systematic studies on tripelennamine or any other H_1-receptor blocker seem to have been performed. Only anecdotal reports on the use of H_2-receptor blockers such as cimetidine have appeared and presently no studies are available to make possible a fair assessment of the value of antihistamines in the treatment of interstitial cystitis.

Sodium Pentosanpolysulfate

The rationale for using sodium pentosanpolysulfate in the treatment of interstitial cystitis was recently reviewed by Parsons (1986, 1987). It is known that the human urothelium has a mucous coat containing polysaccharides (glycosaminoglycans; GAGs) which have been suggested to have an anti-adherence effect important in the bladder's defence against bacteria and toxic agents in the urine. Assuming that patients with interstitial cystitis have a defective or missing surface coat on the urothelium, allowing toxic substances in the urine to penetrate into the bladder and cause an inflammatory reaction, it seems logical to replace the surface polysaccharides with a substitute. The substitute chosen was pentosanpolysulfate (PPS), available in an oral form (Elmiron). It should be stressed, however, that the morphologic appearance of the glycocalyx and of urothelial cells in patients with interstitial cystitis was not different from that of controls (Dixon et al. 1986). This does not exclude qualitative differences in GAG composition (Holm-Bentzen et al. 1986a).

Parsons et al. (1983) reported on the successful treatment of interstitial cystitis patients with PPS. Twenty-four patients with classical symptoms and not responding to intravesical dimethylsulfoxide therapy and/or hydrodistension of the bladder were treated with PPS 50 mg 4 times daily or 150 mg twice daily. Within 4–8 weeks of initiation of treatment 20 patients experienced at least 80% decrease in pain, urgency and nocturia and 2 experienced a 50%–80% decrease in these symptoms. Two patients failed to respond to PPS treatment. Treatment duration was from 6 to 24 months. Parsons (1987) later reported on a placebo-controlled, randomized double-blind study on PPS in interstitial cystitis patients. The patients received 100 mg of PPS 3 times per day or placebo. In these studies, the improvement of pain, urgency, frequency and nocturia were not as impressive as in the initial, open study, but still there was a significant improvement of symptoms in patients receiving PPS.

Other investigators, however, performing controlled clinical studies on the efficacy of PPS in interstitial cystitis reported no superiority over placebo (Squadrito et al. 1985; Holm-Bentzen et al. 1986b; 1987). Presently, the place of PPS in the treatment of interstitial cystitis remains to be established.

Heparin

Theoretically heparin might be effective in the treatment of interstitial cystitis because of its wide range of anti-inflammatory and anti-allergic properties. In addition, it is in part excreted in the urine and may therefore restore a deficient mucous layer in the bladder wall (Lose et al. 1985). Early experiences with systemic and local heparin-treatment were, however, equivocal (Weaver et al. 1963; Badenoch 1971). Lose et al. (1983) reported that 7 patients treated with subcutaneous heparin all had an immediate amelioration of symptoms and an associated fall in elevated levels of eosinophil cationic protein in serum and urine. Lose et al. (1985) found that 6 of 8 patients followed for one year on maintenance injections of heparin (dosage from 5000 units per day to 5000 units 2–3 times per week) continued to experience relief of symptoms. Pelvic pain disappeared within 48 hours of initiation of treatment. Two patients receiving treatment with 5000 units every 4 hours for 2 days followed by 5000 units every 12 hours for 5–7 days required no further therapy.

Although encouraging these reports do not prove the efficacy of heparin in the long-term treatment of interstitial cystitis.

Amitriptyline

Hanno and Wein (1987; 1989) reported that amitriptyline 25–75 mg at bedtime may have beneficial effects in patients with interstitial cystitis. The rationale for the use of this drug is unclear. Hanno and Wein (1987) called for double-blind placebo-controlled trials to establish the efficacy of this drug treatment, but recommended its use in patients refractory to standard treatment (Hanno and Wein 1989).

Dimethyl Sulfoxide (DMSO)

The pharmacology of dimethyl sulfoxide (DMSO) and its application to the treatment of interstitial cystitis was recently reviewed by Sant (1987). DMSO has a wide range of pharmacological effects which theoretically would make it useful for the treatment of interstitial cystitis, including analgesic and anti-inflammatory actions, vasodilatation and dissolution of pathophysiological deposition of collagen. It should be stressed, however, that the mechanism of action of DMSO in interstitial cystitis remains unknown.

Several studies have reported beneficial symptomatic effects of intravesical DMSO in both "early" and "classic" interstitial cystitis. Both adults and children have responded to treatment (Stewart et al. 1972, Stewart and Shirley 1976, Ek et al. 1978; Shirley et al. 1978; Fowler 1981; Biggers 1986; Perez-Marrero et al. 1986, 1988; Barker et al. 1987; Sant 1987). For example, Fowler (1981) treated 20 patients with suspected early interstitial cystitis and achieved complete symptomatic remissions in 3, partial symptomatic remissions in 16, and no effect in 1. Ek et al. (1978) treated 17 patients with Hunner's ulcers and reported an "almost dramatic improvement" in 12. Barker et al. (1987) performed a prospective study of intravesical dimethyl sulfoxide in 30 patients with biopsy-proven chronic inflammatory bladder disease. They reported "satisfactory" symptomatic relief in 80% of the 25 patients who completed treatment.

Most studies performed have been open and without control group. Barker et al. (1987) stressed that the highly characteristic breath, which all their patients experienced for up to 24 hours after the instillation, would preclude any possibility of a "blind" study. However, Perez-Marrero et al. (1986; 1988) reported the results of a placebo-controlled, double-blind cross-over trial involving patients in whom response was assessed both symptomatically and urodynamically. Of patients treated with DMSO 93% had objective improvement compared to 35% of patients receiving placebo. Corresponding figures for subjective improvement were 53% (DMSO) and 18% (placebo).

It has not been settled whether or not DMSO treatment improves the cystoscopic appearance of the bladder. However, in a majority of patients bladder capacity and bladder mucosa remain unchanged (Sant 1987; Barker et al. 1987).

It may be concluded that both open and controlled clinical trials have documented beneficial symptomatic effects of intravesical DMSO in all types of interstitial cystitis. Side effects, local or systemic, have been few and insignificant. Randomized comparisons with other forms of treatment are needed.

Oxychlorosene Sodium (Clorpactin WCS 90)

Oxychlorosene sodium is a mixture of hypochlorous acid and the sodium salt of dodecylbenzene sulfonic acid. The latter component promotes penetration and the germicidal action of the hypochlorite. According to Wishard et al. (1957) the activity of the drug is "dependent upon the liberation of hypochlorous acid and to its oxidating effects, wetting and penetrating properties and detergency". As pointed out by Hanno and Wein (1987) these actions would obviously lead to damage of the bladder luminal mucopolysaccharides, the integrity of which has been postulated to be related to the etiology of the disease.

There are few reported experiences with the drug (Wishard et al. 1957; Murnaghan et al. 1969; Messing and Stamey 1978). Wishard et al. (1957) treated 20 patients with a mean of 5 weekly installations of a 0.2% solution in local anesthesia. Subjective relief was obtained in 14, but cystoscopically signs of interstitial cystitis could still be demonstrated. This contrasts to the findings of

Murnaghan et al. (1969) who treated 17 interstitial cystitis patients according to the protocol of Wishard et al. (1957). They found a positive response in 14 patients and in 10 of these there was associated cystoscopic evidence of healing of the lesions. The duration of satisfactory response extended over several months up to one year. Further courses of treatment were needed by 10 of the 17 patients during an average follow-up of 2 years. Messing and Stamey (1978) reported their experiences of the use of 0.4% solution of oxychlorosene sodium instilled intravesically during full anesthesia in 38 patients with interstitial cystitis. Up to 6 instillations were given, the first 2 at 4-week intervals and the last 4 weekly or every other week. Of the patients, 72% became symptom-free or almost symptom-free for at least 6 months after the final instillation and most of them were asymptomatic for more than one year. The treatment seems to be well tolerated with the exception of irritative symptoms for 1–2 days after the instillation. Ureteral fibrosis has been described as a complication of treatment of a patient with vesicoureteral reflux (Messing and Freiha 1979).

Although published reports are few and controlled clinical trials lacking, oxychlorosene sodium instillations seem to be an effective treatment of interstitial cystitis. Randomized comparisons with other forms of treatment are needed.

Silver Nitrate

Silver nitrate has well known caustic, antiseptic and astringent properties. Its degree of action depends upon the concentration used and the period of time during which the compound is allowed to act. It does not readily penetrate into tissues because the silver ion is precipitated by chloride.

Intravesical instillations of silver nitrate in concentrations up to 2% have for many years been used in the treatment of interstitial cystitis. This obviously non-specific form of therapy has in many studies been combined with hydrodistension and fulguration (Dodson 1926; Pool and Rives 1944; Burford and Burford 1958; Pool 1967; De Juana and Everett 1977). Using instillation of a silver nitrate solution (1 : 2000) as monotherapy, De Juana and Everett (1977) treated 34 patients with mild interstitial cystitis and found a good or excellent one year response in 50%. Sixty-eight patients, presumably with more severe forms of the disease, were treated with silver nitrate in combination with bladder distension and fulguration; 45% had a good or excellent response.

As stated by Messing (1986) most studies on intravesical silver nitrate treatment have used obscure diagnostic and response criteria. A therapeutic effect of silver nitrate cannot be excluded, but its efficacy compared with other forms of treatment remains to be established in controlled trials.

Disodium Cromoglycate

Rosin et al. (1979) investigated 20 histologically proven cases of interstitial cystitis and concluded that it probably is an autoimmune disease. They also induced a chemical cystitis in normal rat bladders and claimed (although no data were provided) that disodium cromoglycate (cromolyn sodium), which is believed to inhibit mediator release from mast cells, had protective properties. Although the possible connection between their findings seemed unclear, Rosin et al. (1979) suggested that sodium cromoglycate may provide a possible means of local treatment of interstitial cystitis. Edwards et al. (1986) presented a hypothesis regarding the etiology of the disease, and reported on 9 patients treated with intravesical instillation of disodium cromoglycate. Six of these responded "satisfactory" to the treatment, whereas 3 derived no benefit. Of the patients responding, one was symptom-free after 2 years, whereas the others still needed regular cystodistension.

Based on available information it cannot be concluded that disodium cromoglycate is an effective treatment of interstitial cystitis.

References

Badenoch AW (1971) Chronic interstitial cystitis. Br J Urol 43:718–721

Barker SB, Mathews PN, Philip PF, Williams G (1987) Prospective study of intravesical dimethyl sulfoxide in the treatment of chronic inflammatory bladder disease. Br J Urol 59:142–144.

Biggers RD (1986) Self-administration of dimethyl sulfoxide (DMSO) for interstitial cystitis. Urology 28:10–11

Burford EH, Burford CE (1958) Hunner's ulcer of the bladder: a report of 187 cases. J Urol 79:952–955

Dees JE (1953) Use of cortisone in interstitial cystitis: preliminary report. J Urol 69:496–502

De Juana CP, Everett Jr JC (1977) Interstitial cystitis: experience and review of recent literature. Urology 10:325–329

Dixon JS, Holm-Bentzen M, Gilpin CJ et al. (1986) Electron microscopic investigation of the bladder urothelium and glycocalyx in patients with interstitial cystitis. J Urol 135:621–625

Dodson AJ (1926) Hunner's ulcer of the bladder; a report of 10 cases. Virginia Med Monthly 53:305–307

Dunn M, Ramsden PD, Roberts JBM, Smith JC, Smith PJB (1977) Interstitial cystitis, treated by prolonged bladder distension. Br J Urol 49:641–645

Edwards L, Bucknall TE, Makin C (1986) Interstitial cystitis: possible cause and clinical study of sodium cromoglycate. Br J Urol 58:95–96.

Ek A, Engberg A, Frodin L, Jonsson G (1978) The use of DMSO in the treatment of interstitial cystitis. Scand J Urol Nephrol 12:129–131

Fall M (1987) Transcutaneous electrical nerve stimulation in interstitial cystitis: update on clinical experience. Urology 29 [Suppl]:40–42

Fall M, Johansson SL, Vahlne A (1985) A clinicopathological and virological study of interstitial cystitis. J Urol 133:771–773

Fall M, Johansson SL, Aldenborg F (1987) Chronic interstitial cystitis: a heterogenous syndrome. J Urol 137:35–38

Fowler JE (1981) Prospective study of intravesical dimethyl sulfoxide in treatment of suspected early interstitial cystitis. Urology 18:21–26

Franksson C (1957) Interstitial cystitis. A clinical study of 59 cases. Acta Chir Scand 113:51–62

Gryglewski RJ (1979) Screening and assessment of the potency of anti-flammatory drugs in vitro. In: Vane JR, Ferreira SH (eds) Anti-inflammatory drugs. Springer, Berlin Heidelberg New York, p 3 (Handbook of experimental pharmacology, vol 50, part 2)

Guerrier HP, Roberts JPM, Slade N (1965) Anti-inflammatory agents in the management of interstitial cystitis. Br J Urol 35:88–92

Hanno PM, Wein AJ (1987) Medical treatment of interstitial cystitis (other than RIMSO-50/Elmiron). Urology 29 [Suppl]:22-26

Hanno PH, Wein AJ (1989) Use of amitriptyline in the treatment of interstitial cystitis. J Urol 141:846–848

Holm-Bentzen M, Ammitzbøll T, Hald T (1986a) Glycosaminoglycans on the surface of the human urothelium: a preliminary report. Neurourol Urodyn 5:519–523

Holm-Bentzen M, Hald T, Larsen S, Jacobsen F, Lose G, Pedersen RH (1986b) A prospective double-blind, clinically controlled multicenter trial of Elmiron in the treatment of painful bladder disease. J Urol 135:187A

Holm-Bentzen M, Jacobson F, Nerstrøm B et al. (1987) A prospective double blind clinically controlled multicenter trial of sodium pentosanpolysulfate in the treatment of interstitial cystitis and related painful bladder disease. J Urol 138:503–507

Holm-Bentzen M, Lose G (1987) Pathology and pathogenesis of interstitial cystitis. Urology 29 [Suppl]:8–13

Hoyt HS (1952) Cortisone in urological conditions with a report of a trial in interstitial cystitis. J Urol 67:899–902

Johnston JH (1956) Local hydrocortisone for Hunner's ulcer of the bladder. Br Med J ii:698–699

Kastrup J, Hald T, Larsen S, Nielsen VG (1983) Histamine content and other types of chronic cystitis. Br J Urol 55:495–500

Kinder CH, Smith RD (1958) Hunner's ulcer. Br J Urol 30:338–343

Larsen S, Thompson SA, Hald T et al. (1982) Mast cells in interstitial cystitis. Br J Urol 54:283–286

Lose G, Frandsen B, Højensgård JC, Jespersen J, Astrup T (1983) Chronic interstitial cystitis: increased levels of eosinophil cationic protein in serum and urine and an ameliorating effect of subcutaneous heparin. Scand J Urol Nephrol 17:159–161

Lose G, Jespersen J, Frandsen B, Højensgård JC, Astrup T (1985) Subcutaneous heparin in the treatment of interstitial cystitis. Scand J Urol Nephrol 19:27–29

Messing EM (1986) Interstitial cystitis and related syndromes. In: Walsh PC et al. (eds) Campbell's urology, 5th edn. Saunders, Philadelphia pp 1070–1086

Messing EM, Freiha FS (1979) Complication of chlorpactin WCS 90 therapy for interstitial cystitis. Urology 13:389–392

Messing EM, Stamey TA (1978) Interstitial cystitis. Early diagnosis, pathology and treatment. Urology 12:381–392

Murnaghan GF, Saalfeld J, Farnsworth RH (1969) Interstitial cystitis – treatment with Chlorpactin WCS 90. Br J Urol 42:744

Oravisto KJ, Alfthan OS (1976) Treatment of interstitial cystitis with immunosuppression and chloroquine derivatives. Eur Urol 2:82–84

Oravisto KJ, Alfthan OS, Jokinen EJ (1970) Interstitial cystitis. Clinical and immunological findings. Scand J Urol Nephrol 4:37–42

Parivar T, Bradbrook RA (1986) Interstitial cystitis. Br J Urol 58:239–244

Parsons CL (1986) Bladder surface glycosaminoglycans: efficient mechanism of environmental adaptation. Urology 27 [Suppl]:9–14

Parsons CL (1987) Sodium pentosanpolysulfate treatment of interstitial cystitis. An update. Urology 29 [Suppl]:14–16

Parsons CL, Schmidt JD, Pollen JJ (1983) Successful treatment of interstitial cystitis with sodium pentosan polysulfate. J Urol 130:51–53

Perez-Marrero R, Emerson LE, Feltis JT (1986) A controlled study of DMSO in interstitial cystitis. J Urol 135:188A

Perez-Marrero R, Emerson LE, Feltis JT (1988) A controlled study of dimethylsulfoxide in interstitial cystitis. J Urol 140:36–39

Pool TL (1967) Interstitial cystitis: clinical considerations and treatment. Clin Obstet Gynecol 10:185

Pool TL, Rives HF (1944) Interstitial cystitis: treatment with silver nitrate. J Urol 51:520–525

Rosin RD, Griffiths T, Sofras F, James DCO, Edwards L (1979) Interstitial cystitis. Br J Urol 51:524–527

Sant GR (1987) Intravesical 50% dimethyl sulfoxide (RIMSO-50) in treatment of interstitial cystitis. Urology 29 [Suppl]:17–21

Shen TY (1979) Prostaglandin synthetase inhibitors I. In: Vane JR, Ferreira SH (eds) Anti-inflammatory drugs. Springer, Berlin Heidelberg New York, p 305 (Handbook of experimental pharmacology, vol 50 part 2)

Shirley SW, Stewart BH, Mirelman S (1978) Dimethyl sulfoxide in treatment of inflammatory genitourinary disorders. Urology 11:215–220

Simmons JL (1961) Interstitial cystitis: an explanation for the beneficial effect of an antihistamine. J Urol 85:149–155

Simmons JL, Bunce PL (1958) On the use of an antihistamine in the treatment of interstitial cystitis. Am Surg 24:664–667

Squadrito JF, Baltish MA, Mullholland SG (1985) Randomized prospective study of sodium pentosan-polysulfate (Elmiron) in treatment of interstitial cystitis. J Urol 133:143A

Stewart BH, Shirley SW (1976) Further experience with intravesical dimethyl sulfoxide in treatment of interstitial cystitis. J Urol 116:36–38

Stewart BH, Branson AC, Hewitt CB, Kiser WS, Straffon RA (1972) The treatment of patients with interstitial cystitis with special reference to intravesical DMSO. J Urol 107:377–380

Walsh A (1978) Interstitial cystitis. In: Harrison JH et al. (eds) Campbell's urology. 4th edn. Saunders, Philadelphia, pp 693–707

Walsh A (1977a) Benzydamine: a new weapon in the treatment of interstitial cystitis. Trans Am Assoc Genito-Urin Surg 68:42

Walsh A (1977b) Interstitial cystitis. Observations on diagnosis and on treatment with anti-inflammatory drugs, particularly benzydamine. Eur Urol 3:216–217

Weaver RG, Dougherty TF, Natoli CA (1963) Recent concepts of interstitial cystitis. J Urol 89:377–383

Wein A (1985) Editorial. Neurourol Urodyn 14:153–155

Wishard Jr WMN, Nourse MH, Mertz JHO (1957) Use of Chlorpactin WCS 90 for relief of symptoms due to interstitial cystitis. J Urol 77:420–423

Chapter 14

Intravesical Therapy of Interstitial Cystitis

P.M. Hanno and A.J. Wein

Despite the multitude of therapies available for the treatment of interstitial cystitis, intravesical lavage with one of a variety of preparations remains the standard treatment against which other treatments must be measured. In this chapter we will review the three most common intravesical treatment medications: silver nitrate, oxychlorosene sodium (Clorpactin WSC-90), and dimethyl sulfoxide.

Silver Nitrate

Pool and Rives (1944) note that the use of silver nitrate can be attributed to Mercier who reported in 1855 that excellent results with bladder instillations had been obtained in patients suffering from symptoms compatible with interstitial cystitis. Dobson in 1926 advocated the use of solutions of silver nitrate in increasing strengths as the treatment of choice for this condition.

In 1944 Pool and Rives reported on 74 patients with interstitial cystitis treated with intravesical silver nitrate. The treatment was carried out as follows:

A urethral catheter is inserted and the contents of the bladder are evacuated. The bladder is then irrigated with a saturated solution of boric acid. Then 30 to 60 cc of a 1 : 5000 solution of silver nitrate is instilled into the bladder and permitted to remain there for 3 or 4 minutes if it does not cause intolerable irritation. At the end of this period the solution is permitted to run out through the catheter, which is then withdrawn. The patient usually experiences some dysuria and vesical irritability for 2 or 3 hours. Treatments are repeated daily unless a severe reaction occurs; in this case, they are repeated every other day. At subsequent treatments, the concentration of silver nitrate in the solution is increased to 1 : 2500, 1 : 1000, 1 : 750, 1 : 500, 1 : 400, 1 : 200, and finally 1 : 100. If at any time the reaction is too severe, the concentration is increased more slowly.

While the initial treatments are performed under general anesthesia, later treatments are given on an outpatient basis. Ureteral reflux would be a contraindication, and it goes without saying that bladder biopsy would be contraindicated just prior to instillation for fear of extravasation. Twenty-three years later, Pool wrote that he still considered this treatment regimen the most efficacious form of treatment (Pool 1967).

The average duration of treatment was 14.2 days. Results were classified as "excellent" in 70% (pain relief, nocturia ×1, daytime frequency every 4 hours) and "good" in 19% (pain relief, nocturia ×3, daytime frequency every 3 hours). The duration of the relief of symptoms varied from 1 to 21 months with an average of 7.6 months.

Hand (1949) used silver nitrate lavage under local anesthesia at varying strengths, usually about 1%. Patients were treated at 6-week intervals. As one of a variety of therapies used in sequence, the results of this modality are not specified in his report.

Burford and Burford (1958) reported on 187 cases of interstitial cystitis treated with silver nitrate. The bladder was locally anesthetized with cocaine hydrochloride and then distended to tolerance. Two percent silver nitrate was then placed into the posterior urethra and vesical neck to which was added 30 ml 1/1000 silver nitrate and 90–120 ml water. The mixture was left in place for 2 minutes and then flushed out with sterile water. The intravesical silver nitrate with or without bladder fulgeration resulted in a 14% "cure" rate and 79% "improved" figure.

Clorpactin WCS 90

O'Conor (1955) reported the use of intravesical Clorpactin WCS 90 at the 1955 meeting of the North Central Section of the American Urological Association. Clorpactin is a generic term for closely related, highly reactive chemical compositions having a modified derivative of hypochlorous acid in a buffered base. Its activity is dependent on the liberation of hypochlorous acid and its resulting oxidizing effects, wetting and penetrating properties, and detergency. Lattimer and Spirito (1955) first used it in the bladder with beneficial results in healing tuberculous ulcers which had not responded to streptomycin para-aminosalicylic acid (PAS) and isonicotinylhydrazine (INH).

Wishard and co-workers (1957) reported on 20 patients with interstitial cystitis who had failed hydrodistention, instillation of silver nitrate, urethral dilatation, anticholinergics, and fulgeration. Clorpactin was administered to each patient from 1 to 10 times with an average total of 5 for each. He describes the procedure in the following way:

2 gm of the powder is dissolved in 1 quart of tepid distilled water. We have always used the solution within an hour or two after it is made up. A catheter is placed in the bladder to empty it. The bladder is then irrigated gently with water after which clorpactin in injected. In patients with a very sensitive bladder only an ounce or two is instilled for a minute. This is withdrawn, the bladder again irrigated with water, and 1 ounce of 2% metycaine instilled in the bladder just before the catheter is withdrawn. In less sensitive patients the bladder is dilated to comfortable capacity with clorpactin, which is then withdrawn. Several such interchanges are used so that the solution is in contact with the bladder for 3–5 minutes. The treatments are repeated weekly for a total of 5.

Of Wishard's 20 patients, 14 reported subjective improvement.

Murnaghan and colleagues (1970) treated 17 patients according to the above protocol and noted significant improvement in 14 patients. Ten patients required further treatment during the average 2-year follow-up.

Messing and Stamey (1978) reported on the use of 0.4% solution of Clorpactin WCS 90 on 38 patients, noting a 72% success rate in achieving an almost symptom-free state for at least 6 months. Full anesthesia was required because of extreme pain on instillation. Instillations were given weekly, with a one month pause after the first 2 instillations to await a therapeutic response. A case of ureteral fibrosis complicating the treatment prompted the recommendation that vesicoureteral reflux be considered a contraindication to the procedure (Messing and Freiha 1979).

Dimethyl Sulfoxide (DMSO)

The mainstay of treatment for interstitial cystitis is the intravesical instillation of dimethyl sulfoxide (DMSO). DMSO is a product of the wood pulp industry and a derivative of lignin. It has exceptional solvent properties and is freely miscible with water, lipids, and organic agents. Pharmacologic properties include membrane penetration, enhanced drug absorption, anti-inflammatory, analgesic, collagen dissolution, muscle relaxant, and mast cell histamine-release. Tests for DMSO for treatment of human illness began in the 1960s in the areas of musculoskeletal inflammation and the cutaneous manifestations of scleroderma. Sant recently published a comprehensive summary of DMSO in the treatment of interstitial cystitis (Sant 1987).

Stewart is responsible for popularizing intravesical DMSO for interstitial cystitis. In the mid 1960s he applied it to the skin over the suprapubic area in a group of patients refractory to conventional forms of therapy. It was hoped that its deep penetrating properties and primarily urinary excretion would allow for a beneficial response. Only 2 of 15 patients improved. Stewart went on to test intravesical delivery of 50 ml of a 50% solution instilled for 15 minutes by urinary catheter. Treatments were repeated at intervals of 2–4 weeks depending on therapeutic response. Six of the first 8 patients reported significant symptomatic relief lasting 2–12 months in the initial report (Stewart et al. 1967) The lack of side-effects (other than a garlic-like odor on the breath) or need for inpatient administration were significant breakthroughs over previous treatments.

Because of possible ophthalmic toxicity in animals receiving large oral doses of DMSO, the drug was withdrawn by the US Government from further human study in the late 1960s. Animal studies confirmed the safety of intravesical administration, and further patient trials were instituted and reported by Stewart in 1971. Twelve of 21 patients had good to excellent results, with good defined as 1 month symptom-free after instillation, and excellent 3 months symptom-free after instillation. Follow-up cystoscopy did not reveal any change in bladder appearance in most patients.

Five years later Stewart (1976) summarized his experience with intravesical DMSO in 46 patients treated at bi-weekly intervals until symptoms responded, with treatment intervals then adjusted appropriately based on length of response. Good or excellent responses occured in 73% of patients, i.e. patients were relatively free of symptoms at least 1–3 months between instillations. In a later report Stewart's group (Shirley et al. 1978) recommended intravesical

DMSO therapy for a variety of other conditions including radiation cystitis, chronic prostatitis, and refractory chronic female trigonitis. He stressed the absence of systemic or local toxicity in 213 patients.

Ek et al. (1978) reported a 70% success rate, but found most patients ultimately required retreatment or further therapy with other modalities. Prospective series of Fowler (1981) and Barker et al. (1987) revealed symptomatic success rates of greater than 80%, although relapse was not uncommon. Fowler noted only minimal improvements in functional bladder capacity, and attributed the beneficial effects of DMSO to a direct effect on the sensory nerves of the bladder. In an interesting study, Emerson and Feltis (1986) showed that patients with bladder instability and symptoms of interstitial cystitis fail to respond to intravesical DMSO, making the diagnosis at least suspect in patients with uninhibited contractions on urodynamic evaluation.

With its ease of administration (Biggers 1986), lack of side effects, and dependable symptomatic results, DMSO certainly merits its place as one of the first-line treatments for this difficult and often frustrating condition. Our group has been adding 5000 units of heparin to the DMSO, mainly on theoretical grounds. Studies suggest the compound's ability to mimic the activity of the bladder's own mucopolysaccharide lining (Hanno et al. 1978). In addition, heparin has anti-inflammatory effects as well as actions which inhibit fibroblast proliferation, angiogenesis, and smooth muscle cell proliferation (Trelstad 1985). Weaver injected heparin transcystoscopically and used it as an intravesical lavage in 7 patients with good results, though follow-up was brief (Weaver et al. 1963). Studies from Scandinavia have suggested beneficial effects of systemically administered heparin (Lose et al. 1983, 1985), though the most recent report shows subcutaneous heparin no better than placebo in a controlled study of 39 patients (Holm-Bentzen et al. 1988). Our results with a mixture of heparin and DMSO administered intravesically appear to be no better than results in the literature for DMSO used alone. A prospective double-blind trial would be necesssary to determine if heparin has any place whatever in the treatment of interstitial cystitis.

References

Barker SB, Matthews PN, Philip PF, Williams G (1987) Prospective study of intravesical dimethyl sulphoxide in the treatment of chronic inflammatory bladder disease. Br J Urol 59:142–144

Biggers RD (1986) Self-administration of dimethyl sulfoxide (DMSO) for interstitial cystitis. Urology 28:10–11

Burford EH, Burford CE (1958) Hunner's ulcer of the bladder: a report of 187 cases. J Urol 79:952–955

Dodson AI (1926) Hunner's ulcer of the bladder; a report of ten cases. Va Med Mon 53:305–310

Ek A, Engberg A, Frodin L Jonsson G (1978) The use of dimethyl sulfoxide (DMSO) in the treatment of interstitial cystitis. Scand J Urol Nephrol 12:129–131

Emerson LE, Feltis JT (1986) Urodynamic factors affecting response to DMSO in patients with interstitial cystitis. J Urol 135:188A

Fowler JE (1981) Prospective study of intravesical dimethyl sulfoxide in treatment of suspected early interstitial cystitis. Urology 28:21–26

Hand JR (1949) Interstitial cystitis: report of 223 cases (204 women and 19 men). J Urol 61:291–310

Hanno PM, Fritz R, Wein AJ et al. (1978) Heparin as antibacterial agent in rabbit bladder. Urology 12:411–415

Holm-Bentzen M, Lose G, Frandsen B et al. (1988) A clinically controlled double-blind study of subcutaneous heparin in the treatment of interstitial cystitis. J Urol 139:227A

Lattimer JK, Spirito AL (1955) Clorpactin for tuberculous cystitis. J Urol 73:1015–1018

Lose G, Frandsen B, Højensgård JC et al. (1983) Chronic interstitial cystitis: increased levels of eosinophil cationic protein in serum and urine and an ameliorating effect of subcutaneous heparin. Scand J Urol Nephrol 17:159–161

Lose G, Jespersen J, Frandsen B et al. (1985) Subcutaneous heparin in the treatment of interstitial cystitis. Scand J Urol Nephrol 19:27–29

Messing EM, Freiha FS (1979) Complication of clorpactin WCS 90 therapy for interstitial cystitis. Urology 13:389–392

Messing EM, Stamey TA (1978) Interstitial cystitis, early diagnosis, pathology, and treatment. Urology 12:381–392

Murnaghan GF, Saalfeld J, Farnsworth RH (1970) Interstitial cystitis – treatment with chlorpactin WCS 90. Br J Urol 42:744

O'Conor VJ (1955) Clorpactin WCS 90 in the treatment of interstitial cystitis. Q Bull NWU Med Sch 29:392

Pool TL (1967) Interstitial cystitis: clinical considerations and treatment. Clin Obstet Gynecol 10:185–191

Pool TL, Rives HF (1944) Interstitial cystitis: treatment with silver nitrate. J Urol 51:520–525

Sant GR (1987) Intravesical 50% dimethyl sulfoxide (rimso-50) in treatment of interstitial cystitis. Urology [Suppl] 29:17–21

Shirley SW, Stewart BH, Mirelman S (1978) Dimethyl sulfoxide in treatment of inflammatory genitourinary disorders. Urology 11:215–220

Stewart BH, Shirley SW (1976) Further experience with intravesical dimethyl sulfoxide in the treatment of interstitial cystitis. J Urol 116:36–38

Stewart BH, Persky L, Kiser WS (1967) The use of dimethyl sulfoxide (DMSO) in the treatment of interstitial cystitis. J Urol 98:671–672

Stewart BH, Branson AC, Hewitt CB, Kiser WS, Straffon RA (1971) The treatment of patients with interstitial cystitis, with special reference to intravesical DMSO. Trans Am Assoc Genitourin Surg 63:69–72

Trelstad RL (1985) Glycosaminoglycans: mortar, matrix, mentor. Lab Invest 53:1–4

Weaver RG, Dougherty TF, Natoli CA (1963) Recent concepts of interstitial cystitis. J Urol 89:377–383

Wishard WN, Nourse MH, Mertz JHO (1957) Use of clorpactin WCS 90 for relief of symptoms due to interstitial cystitis. J Urol 77:420–423

Chapter 15

Subcutaneous Heparin in the Treatment of Interstitial Cystitis

G. Lose and B. Fransden

Due to elusive etiology and pathogenesis the treatment of interstitial cystitis (IC) has hitherto been empirical. Although the therapeutic modalities have been numerous, ranging from what is truly homeopathic to major surgery, the treatment of this distressing chronic inflammatory condition of the bladder remains difficult and laborious. New knowledge, however, concerning the inflammatory process of the bladder wall has offered more rational avenues of treatment. Recent histopathological studies have shown increased mast cell density, degranulation and infiltration of eosinophils in the bladder wall in patients with IC (Larsen et al. 1982; Fall et al. 1985; Aldenborg et al. 1986; Lose et al. 1987; Lynes et al. 1987). Furthermore, chemical mediators, or their metabolites, originating from mast cells and eosinophils have been found in the bladder wall and in urine from IC patients (Kastrup et al. 1983; Holm-Bentzen et al. 1987; Lose et al. 1987). These findings parallel observations performed in other chronic inflammatory conditions such as Crohn's disease (Binder 1979; Dvorak 1979) and ulcerative proctocolitis (Binder 1979; Heatley et al. 1979).

Mast cells and eosinophils play a central role in the normal inflammatory response which aids in the elimination of microorganisms or toxic agents. However, they seem also intimately involved in the complicated cellular and biochemical interactions of various pathological or "unregulated" conditions which may lead to allergic reactions or chronic inflammation with tissue destruction and fibrosis (Wasserman 1979). The latter seems to be the pathogenesis in different chronic inflammatory diseases such as IC. Therefore, a rational therapeutic approach seems to be pharmacologic interruption or damping of the inflammatory process in the bladder wall.

For this purpose heparin treatment seems rational. Heparin belongs to the class of linear anionic polyelectrolytes, which possesses a wide range of biological activities, the anticoagulant activity being the most established. However, heparin may also:

1. Exert a membrane-stabilizing effect on mast cells (Jaques 1978)
2. Antagonize histamine, bradykinin and prostaglandin E_1 (Carr 1979)
3. Inhibit the complement system and the action of inflammatory hormones (Jaques 1980)

4. Inhibit fibroblast proliferation, angiogenesis and smooth muscle proliferation (Trelstad 1985)

In addition, heparin, which is a glycosoaminoglycan, is in part excreted in the urine (Jaques 1980), and it may therefore restore a deficient mucous layer of the bladder wall which has been demonstrated in animal experiments (Hanno et al. 1978). Heparin also seems to play an important role in the physiological repair of injuries to tissues of the body (Saliba et al. 1973). In some patients with IC this process of tissue repair may be defective due to excessive formation of fibrin which may lead to extensive fibrosis and scar formation (Kwaan and Astrup 1964). This may explain why some patients develop a small contracted bladder. Heparin may prevent this sequence by reducing the deposition of fibrin sufficient for premature hemostasis and wound healing.

Administration and Dose

We have used subcutaneous administration of heparin in the treatment of IC beginning with 5000 IU every 8 hours for 2 days, followed by 5000 IU every 12 hours for 5–14 days (Lose et al. 1983, 1985). After this initial administration, the treatment is discontinued. If symptoms recur the administration of heparin is resumed and continued by self-administration after discharge from hospital, using disposable syringes continuing 5000 IU of heparin in 0.2 ml. The maintenance dose is individualized ranging from 5000 per day to 5000 IU 2–3 times per week.

Side Effects

Side effects have not been observed, in particular no cases of spontaneous hemorrhage. Menstrual bleeding, however, may be increased.

Comments

Heparin treatment of IC was introduced more than 20 years ago (Kárpáti 1964; Weaver et al. 1963). Both Weaver et al. (1963) and Kárpáti (1964) combined local application of heparin with a short (3–4 days) intravenous adminstration. We have chosen the subcutaneous administration because of the simplicity and safeness of this method. Furthermore, this method permits the patients to perform self-administration. The dose used increases the activated partial thromboplastin time up to 10%, but we do not routinely measure coagulation parameters.

Until now we have treated, or been involved in the treatment of, about 30 patients. Our preliminary results in small groups of selected patients (Lose et al. 1983, 1985) have been promising enough to initiate an ongoing controlled study.

In typical cases bladder pain disappears within 24–48 hours after therapy has been initiated. The effect on frequency depends on the capacity of the bladder. Due to this pattern of response, and according to previous reports, we have kept the initial treatment short (maximum 2 weeks). However, it is an open question whether extended treatment may have an effect in patients without response within one month. Some concern has been expressed regarding possible effects of long-term heparin treatment (Jaques 1980).

In some non-responders we have combined the subcutaneous treatment with local instillation in the bladder of heparin. In these cases we have used 50 000 IU heparin dissolved in 10 ml sterile saline. This solution is left in the bladder until the next voiding. This treatment has also been used successfully in other cases of painful bladder disease, e.g. radiation cystitis.

According to our experience symptoms often reappear within one month after discontinuation of the initial treatment. In these patients it is normally possible to obtain a persistent effect on a maintenance dose. We routinely try to discontinue treatment every 3 months. There seems to be a cumulative effect of long-term treatment leading to increased length of periods without symptoms after discontinuation of treatment.

The results obtained with subcutaneous heparin are in agreement with the results reported by Parsons who used a low molecular weight heparin-like compound (Elmiron) administered orally (Parsons et al. 1983).

Although there have at the present time been no controlled studies documenting the effect of subcutaneous heparin in patients with IC, this treatment has been promising and seems rational according to current hypotheses concerning etiology and pathogenesis (Holm-Bentzen and Lose 1987).

References

Aldenborg F, Fall M, Enerbäck L (1986) Proliferation and transepithelial migration of mucosal mast cells in interstitial cystitis. Immunology 58:411–416

Binder V (1979) Eosinophilia in chronic inflammatory bowel disease. Does it reflect activity or pathogenesis? In: Pepys J, Edwards AM (eds) The mast cell. Pitman Medical, London, pp 668–672

Carr J (1979) The anti-inflammatory action of heparin. Heparin as an antagonist to histamine, bradykinin and prostaglandin E_1. Thromb Res 16:507–516

Dvorak AM (1979) Mast-cell hyperlasia and degranulation in Crohn's disease. In: Pepys J, Edwards AM (eds) The mast cell. Pitman Medical, London, pp 657–662

Fall M, Aldenborg F, Enerbäck L, Johansson SL (1985) Interstitial cystitis is two diseases. Proceedings of the 15th annual meeting of the ICS, London, pp 250–251

Hanno PM, Fritz R, Wein AJ, Mulholland SG (1978) Heparin as antibacterial agent in rabbit bladder. Urology 12:411–415

Heatley RV, James PD, Birkinshaw M, Wenham RB, Mayberry J, Rhodes (1979) The role of interstitial mast cells and eosinophil cells in ulcerative proctocolitis in relation to prognosis and treatment. In: Pepys J, Edwards AM (eds) The mast cells. Pitman Medical, London, pp 716–724.

Holm-Bentzen M, Lose G (1987) Pathology and pathogenesis of interstitial cystitis. Urology 29 [Suppl]:8–13

Holm-Bentzen M, Søndergaard I, Hald T (1987) Urinary excretion of a metabolite of histamine (1,4-methyl-imidazole-acetic acid) in painful bladder disease. Br J Urol 59:230–233

Jaques LB (1978) Endogenous Heparin. Semin Thromb Haemost 4:326–349

Jaques LB (1980) Heparins: anionic polyelectrolyte drugs. Pharmacol Rev 31:99–167

Kárpáti F (1964) Behandlung des ulcus simplex vesicae urinariae (Hunnersches Geschwür) mit heparin. Z Urol 12:895–898

Kastrup J, Hald T, Larsen S, Nielsen VG (1983) Histamine content and mast cell count of detrusor muscle in patients with interstitial cystitis and other types of chronic cystitis. Br J Urol 55: 495–500

Kwaan HC, Astrup T (1964) Fibrinolytic activity of reparative connective tissue. J Pathol Bacteriol 87:409–414

Larsen S, Thompson SA, Hald T et al. (1982) Mast cells in interstitial cystitis. Br J Urol 54:283–286

Lose G, Frandsen B, Højensgård JC, Jespersen J, Astrup T (1983) Chronic interstitial cystitis: increased levels of eosinophil cationic protein in serum and urine and an ameliorating effect of subcutaneous heparin. Scand J Urol Nephrol 17:159–161

Lose G, Jespersen J, Frandsen B, Højensgård JC, Astrup T (1985) Subcutaneous heparin in the treatment of interstitial cystitis. Scand J Urol Nephrol 19:27–29

Lose G, Frandsen B, Holm-Bentzen M, Larsen S, Jacobsen F (1987) Urine eosinophil cationic protein in painful bladder disease. Br J Urol 60:39–42

Lynes WL, Flynn SD, Shortliffe LD et al. (1987) Mast cell involvement in interstitial cystitis. J Urol 138:746–751

Parsons CL, Schmidt JD, Polen JJ (1983) Successful treatment of interstitial cystitis with sodium pentosanpolysulfate. J Urol 130:51–53

Saliba Jr MJ, Dempsey WC, Kruggel JL (1973) Large burns in humans. Treatment with heparin. JAMA 225:261–269

Trelstad RL (1985) Glycosaminoglycans: mortar, matrix, mentor. Lab Invest 53:1–4

Wasserman SI (1979) The mass cell and the inflammatory response. In: Pepys J, Edwards AM (eds) The mast cell. Pitman Medical, London, pp 9–20

Weaver RG, Dougherty TF, Natoli CA (1963) Recent concepts of interstitial cystitis. J Urol 89:377–383

Chapter 16

Urine Eosinophil Cationic Protein in Painful Bladder Disease

G. Lose and B. Fransden

Hitherto, no blood or urine analyses have been encountered which provide specific diagnostic information to classify patients with painful bladder disease. However, we have observed an increased level of eosinophil cationic protein in urine (U-ECP) in patients with interstitial cystitis (IC) (Lose et al. 1983, 1988) and recently it has been shown that these patients also have elevated urinary excretion of metabolites of histamine (Holm-Bentzen et al. 1987).

Eosinophil Cationic Protein (ECP)

ECP has been isolated from human eosinophils and constitutes 30% of the protein of the eosinophil granules (Olsson and Venge 1974). It is a highly cationic zinc containing single-chained protein with a molecular weight of about 20 000 (Venge et al. 1980; Lose et al. 1987). ECP seems to be involved in the regulation of the humoral part of inflammation by modulation of coagulation, fibrinolysis and the kallikrein–kinin system (Venge et al. 1980). It has also proven toxic against many cells and tissues (Frigas et al. 1980; Tai et al. 1982, 1984).

We have developed an enzyme immunoassay based on antigen obtained from patients with IC, for the determination of ECP in urine. In healthy individuals we have estimated a normal range of 18–32 arb. U/l (Frandsen and Lose 1986) and less than 36 arb. U/l in patients with irritative voiding symptoms but a normal bladder biopsy (Lose et al. 1987).

ECP and IC

Histopathologic studies have shown increased mast cell density, mast cell degranulation and infiltrations of eosinophils in the bladder wall in patients with

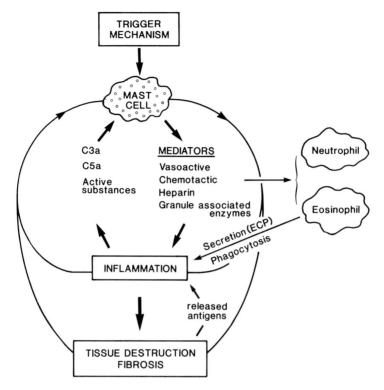

Fig. 16.1. Schematic representation of some inflammatory events possibly involved in the pathogenesis of interstitial cystitis.

IC. It is suggested that the inflammatory process in the bladder wall is triggered by some noxious agent (in urine or blood) or caused by a defective local defence mechanism against components in urine which may activate (immunologically or non-immunologically) mast cells. This subsequently leads to release of chemical mediators including histamine which provokes an inflammatory response characterized among other things by vasodilation, smooth muscle contraction, increased vascular permeability, chemotaxis of eosinophils and neutrophils and complement activation. The attracted eosinophils modify the inflammatory response through deposition of granule products including ECP and/or phagocytosis of mast cell products. These inflammatory events probably play a central role in normal homeostasis by eliminating microorganisms or toxic agents but may, if "unregulated" lead to tissue destruction, chronic inflammation and fibrosis (Wasserman 1979). Eosinophil secretion of ECP is suggested to enhance the generation of substances that potentiate the inflammatory response which may be beneficial, in parasite infections for example, but may have an aggravating effect in various inflammatory diseases (Dahl 1979) and therefore may play a role in the pathogenesis of IC, by stimulating a circulus vitiosus (Fig. 16.1).

Generally patients with IC do not have peripheral eosinophilia. However, in patients with IC according to the histopathological criteria of Larsen el al. (1982) we have revealed a highly significant increased median level of U-ECP, 140

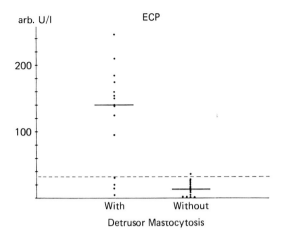

Fig. 16.2. Urinary concentration of eosinophil cationic protein (ECP) in 30 patients with painful bladder disease (15 with and 15 without detrusor mastocytosis). Median values are shown and the normal range upper limit indicated by the *dashed line*. (Reproduced with permission from Lose et al. (1987) Br J Urol 60:39–42).

arb.U/l versus 14 arb.U/l in patients with normal histology (Fig. 16.2). Since ECP is unable to pass beyond the kidney (Venge, personal communication), it is suggested that the increased concentration in urine in patients with IC originates from the local inflammatory process in the bladder wall. Our observations of a high rate of eosinophil infiltrations in the biopsies and a negative correlation between U-ECP and the number of blood eosinophils in patients with IC indicate that eosinophils are attracted to the inflammatory site and stimulated in situ to release their granule contents (Lose et al. 1987). It is possible that ECP may be responsible for the damage to the bladder leading to fibrosis. Recently we have found in in vitro studies that ECP in concentrations found in urine have immediate as well as late effects on kidney epithelium cells. The immediate effects observed were detachment of cells from the epithelium and a cytotoxic effect. After 24 hours a dose-related stimulation of cell proliferation was observed.

Comments

Measurement of U-ECP has provided a new tool to study patients with painful bladder disease. Elevated U-ECP is closely correlated with an increased number of mast cells in the detrusor muscle and therefore can be used to select patients with IC according to criteria of Larsen et al. (1982). We have observed, however, that U-ECP may be significantly elevated in patients with tuberculosis and cancer in the bladder, whereas in acute bacterial cystitis U-ECP may be normal or slightly elevated. U-ECP probably may be useful in screening patients with painful bladder disease and in monitoring the effect of treatment. Thus, we have observed a close correlation between improvement of the clinical symptoms and decrease of U-ECP during treatment with heparin (Lose et al.

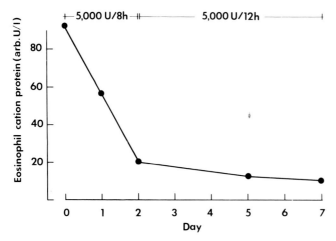

Fig. 16.3. The concentration of ECP in urine during successful treatment with subcutaneous heparin in a patient with IC.

1983) (Fig. 16.3). This may be due to neutralization of ECP, restoration of a defect layer in glycosaminoglycans in the bladder or to less specific anti-inflammatory effects of heparin. In patients with chronic bowel disease, tissue infiltration with eosinophils has been suggested to provide information concerning activity of the disease and the prognosis (Heatley et al. 1979). In IC elevated U-ECP is often associated with severe symptoms and may reflect activity of the disease, whereas the correlation between ECP and the prognosis remains elusive.

References

Dahl R (1979) The eosinophil cell and eosinophil cationic protein in bronchial asthma. In: Pepys J, Edwards AM (eds) The mast cell. Pitman Medical, London, pp 101–105

Frandsen B, Lose G (1986) Determination of eosinophil cationic protein in urine by an enzyme immunoassay. Scand J Clin Lab Invest 46:629–634.

Frigas E, Loegering DA, Gleich DA, Gleich GJ (1980) Cytotoxic effects of the guinea pig eosinophil major basic protein on tracheal epithelium. Lab Invest 42:35–43.

Heatley RV, James PD, Birkinshaw M, Wenham RB, Mayberry J, Rhodes J (1979) The role of interstitial mast cells and eosinophil cells in ulcerative proctocolitis in relation to prognosis and treatment. In: Pepys J, Edwards AM (eds) The mast cell. Pitman Medical, London, pp 716–724

Holm-Bentzen M, Søndergaard I, Hald T (1987) Urinary excretion of a metabolite of histamine (1,4-methyl-imidazole-acetic acid) in painful bladder disease. Br J Urol 59:230–233

Larsen S, Thompson SA, Hald T et al. (1982) Mast cells in interstitial cystitis. Br J Urol 54:283–286

Lose G, Frandsen B, Højensgård JC, Jespersen J, Astrup T (1983) Chronic interstitial cystitis: increased levels of eosinophil cationic protein in serum and urine and an ameliorating effect of subcutaneous heparin. Scand J Urol Nephrol 17:159–161

Lose G, Frandsen B, Holm-Bentzen M, Larsen S, Jacobsen F (1987) Urine eosinophil cationic protein in painful bladder disease. Br J Urol 60:39–42

Olsson I, Venge P (1974) Cationic proteins of human granulocytes. II. Separation of the cationic proteins of the granules of leukemic myeloid cells. Blood 44:235–246.

Tai P-C, Hayes DJ, Clark JB, Spry CJF (1982) Toxic effects of human eosinophil secretion products on isolated rat heart cells in vitro. Biochem J 204:75–80

Tai P-C, Holt ME, Denny P, Gibbs AR, Williams BD, Spry CJF (1984) Disposition of eosinophil cationic protein in granulomas in allergic granulomatosis and vasculitis: the Churg-Strauss syndrome. Br Med J 289:400–402

Venge P, Dahl R, Hällgren, Olsson I (1980) Cationic proteins of the human eosinophils and their role in the inflammatory reaction. In: Mahmoud AAF, Austen KF (eds) The eosinophil in health and disease. Grune and Stratton, New York, pp 131–142

Wasserman SI (1979) The mast cell and the inflammatory response. In: Pepys J, Edwards AM (eds) The mast cell. Pitman Medical, London, pp 9–20

Chapter 17

Use of Pentosanpolysulfate in the Management of Interstitial Cystitis

C.L. Parsons

The pathogenesis of interstitial cystitis is currently unknown. One possible etiology is that the transitional epithelium is defective, leading to molecular leaks that initiate the disease complex. This theory was the principle rationale for the employment by us of pentosanpolysulfate (PPS) in the therapy of interstitial cystitis.

In the past 10 years, a series of ongoing experiments has demonstrated that an important cell surface defense mechanism of the transitional epithelium is the surface polysaccharide, or glycosaminoglycans (GAG). An intact glycosamino-glycan layer acts as an effective barrier that prevents the adherence of bacteria, microcrystals, proteins and ions (Parsons 1982; Parsons et al. 1975, 1977, 1980a, 1980b, 1985; Gill et al. 1982). This important cell surface defense mechanism can be injured with protamine-like substances which impair anti-adherent activity and allow increased adherence of potentially harmful substances such as microcrystals, proteins or calcium (Parsons et al. 1981, 1988; Kaufman et al. 1987). In addition, protamine sulfate has been found to greatly alter the permeability of the cell surface to an uncharged molecule, urea (Parsons et al. 1990). This is an important observation since it demonstrates that alteration of the cell surface glycosaminoglycans can lead to a leak. This is the first model which has demonstrated that such a phenomenon could occur.

A preliminary study was done to determine whether a sulfated poly-saccharide, pentosanpolysulfate, could alleviate the symptom complex associated with interstitial cystitis. In the pilot study (Parsons et al. 1983), 90% of the patients reported amelioration of their symptoms while taking the medication. The rationale for using such a substance was to attempt to place at the bladder surface, a more anti-adherent compound that is naturally present (it is more highly sulfated than native polysaccharide) which could potentially block leaks (occurring for whatever reason). In addition, in view of the fact that protamine sulfate-like compounds present in the urine could potentially damage bladder surface polysaccharide, it was felt that by placing a drug such as pentosanpolysulfate into the urine, it could scavenge and detoxify protamine-like substances.

Summarized here will be the results of two controlled studies to evaluate the effect on interstitial cystitis of pentosanpolysulfate administered either orally or parenterally.

Materials and Methods

Patients

The patients had to have the syndrome of frequency, urgency, nocturia, and/or pain and the absence of negative urine cultures, negative cytologies and negative biopsies where appropriate (those patients suspected of having carcinoma on cystoscopy). To qualify for the studies they had to void a minimum of 8 times per day, average more than one void per night and complain of moderate urinary urgency. The symptom complex had to be continuously present for at least one year. All patients had cystoscopy performed when they were symptomatic and only those individuals showing a bladder capacity of less than 900 ml and either a Hunner's ulcer or petechial hemorrhages after hydrodistension, were included.

Patients were entered into the study after one month had elapsed following endoscopic evaluation. This was to prevent any beneficial effects of the hydrodistension from raising placebo response rate.

The functional voiding capacity was obtained by doing a micturitional profile of the patients over 3 days during which time the patients recorded all the voids in terms of both time and amount.

The patient's subjective parameters were obtained by asking them to complete a form in which they recorded their impression of their frequency and nocturia and rated their pain and urgency on a 4-point scale. At subsequent visits, the patients would again record their concept of their frequency, nocturia and any improvement they felt in urgency or pain on a 5-point scale (0%–100% improvement). In addition, they would record on a 5-point scale the percentage of overall improvement they felt since the onset of therapy (0%, 25%, 50%, 75% 100%). At the follow-up visits the patients also provided micturitional profiles for evaluation.

Successful management was defined prior to the study. Patients had to report a greater than 25% overall improvement, an average of at least 3 fewer voids per day, and an average increase of at least 10 ml per void. The same was true of the pain and urgency scales: patients had to report a greater than 25% improvement. In the subsequent study with subcutaneous administration of the medication, there was an additional scale of pain and urgency added where the patients recorded their pain and urgency on a scale of 1–10 and did so at all subsequent visits. This was not done for the initial oral study.

Oral Study

When the patients had filled out all their data sheets and completed their cystoscopic evaluations, they were randomized in double-blind fashion to either drug or placebo. The individuals in the drug group received 100 mg pentosanpolysulfate 3 times per day. Patients were initially randomized and put into treatment arm A. They were monitored at 3-month intervals and if during the course of two follow-up visits they had continuous improvement of the symptoms, they were considered to be successfully treated (this required at least a 37.5% or better improvement) and completed the study. Those patients who showed no response at the end of 3 months of therapy, were crossed over from whatever treatment they were receiving to the other arm of the study (treatment arm B).

Subcutaneous Therapy

Patients who entered a later study for subcutaneous therapy were evaluated prior to entry in a manner identical to the patients in the oral study. The only difference was that the scale used for these patients to evaluate pain and urgency was a 10-point scale, 10 being the worst pain. In addition, the duration of the study was 12 weeks and they were evaluated at the beginning and at the end of the study following randomization to either drug or placebo. The patients received either 100 mg of either pentosanpolysulfate or saline on Monday, Wednesday, and Friday. They were randomized in a double-blind fashion.

Results

Studying interstitial cystitis would appear superficially to be a difficult problem, but if the study is set up right, definitions of success are made prior to commencement of the study, and one looks at the percentage of patients achieving significant improvements, it is relatively easy to see whether the therapy is successful. One can monitor any symptom, pain, urgency, or overall improvement, and see it reflected in the micturitional profile. The most useful parameter remained the overall improvement that the patients subjectively felt, as it correlated with (Parsons et al. 1983) improvements in all subjective and objective parameters obtained.

Patients receiving oral PPS reported a 47% overall improvement of their symptom complex as opposed to only 23% of the placebo patients ($P < 0.05$). Patients receiving the drug did significantly better than those receiving placebo whether one looked at either subjective or objective data as recorded in the micturitional profiles (see Tables 17.1 and 17.2). One important aspect of the study was, as noted above, that if a patient reported a significant overall improvement (whether on drug or placebo), it was discovered that there was improvement in all that patient's subjective and objective parameters. Those who reported no improvement, whether on drug or placebo, had no improvement in any of their subjective or objective parameters. The important point is that one should define criteria for success for each parameter prior to the onset of study and look at the percentage of patients satisfying those criteria, rather than taking a simple mean for the whole group. This is important because to put patients with very severe disease, who do worse in general, into studies such as this can obscure successful management of those patients with more moderate disease.

Table 17.1. Results of four symptoms evaluated for all patients

	Placebo	Drug	P value
Pain			
No. improved/total (%)	7/38 (18)	19/42 (45)	0.02
Average % improvement*	15.8 ± 26	33.0 ± 35	0.01
Urgency			
No. improved/total (%)	9/48 (19)	21/42 (40)	0.03
Average % improvement*	14.0 ± 24	27.6 ± 31	0.01
Frequency			
No. improved/total (%)	16/41 (39)	33/52 (63)	0.005
Average improvement	−0.4	−5.1	0.002
Nocturia			
Average improvement[a]	−0.5 ± 0.5	−1.5 ± 2.9	0.04

In all parameters the drug did significantly better than placebo. Responses were considered good only if the patient experienced at least 50% improvement. For pain and urgency, each patient reported the average percentage improvement that they experienced, and the value presented represents the average improvements noted for these symptoms for all patients in the group. Frequency results are reported as the percentage of patients with any improvement and as the average change reported by the patient after therapy. *P* values were obtained by comparing placebo with drug. Each group represents the patients who started on a treatment arm or were crossed over to an arm, such that some patients were on both arms.

[a] Mean ± standard deviation.

Table 17.2. Average number of daily voids and bladder volumes determined by micturitional profiles

	Placebo	Drug
No. of patients	29	34
Average no. daily voids[a]		
Before therapy	20.1 ± 9	18.9 ± 9
After therapy	20.8 ± 13*	18.3 ± 10**
Net difference	0.7	−0.6
No. improved%	6 (21)	13 (38)
Average voided volume (ml)[b]		
Before therapy	80.4 ± 42	85.2 ± 46
After therapy	84.6 ± 53**	102.5 ± 57***
Average change	4.2	17.3

P values were determined by Student's *t* test. Each group represents the patients who were evaluated after cross-over, such that some received drug and placebo therapy.

[a] Net difference represents the difference in voids per day before and after therapy. Number improved is the number of subjects with at least 3 fewer voids per day. With regard to this factor the drug did better than the placebo ($P = 0.1$).
[b] There was a significant increase in bladder capacity in the drug group ($P = 0.009$), but not in the placebo group.
* $P = 0.6$; ** $P = 0.5$; *** $P = 0.009$.

For the patients who received injectable therapy, there was significant overall improvement noted in 50% of patients on drug and a 14% improvement in the placebo group. These differences were highly significant ($P < 0.02$). Thus, in the oral studies the patients on drug did better in both their subjective and objective parameters than patients on placebo (see Tables 17.1 and 17.2). One difference seen between the injection versus the oral medication was that injected patients started to report significant improvements as early as 2–3 weeks as opposed to 4–6 weeks in the patients receiving oral therapy.

Comments

While we selected PPS as a potential therapy for this disease for the rationale described above, i.e. to provide the surface with a more sulfated polysaccharide or to scavenge urinary protamine-like substances, I would like to emphasize that we do not necessarily think that patients with this symptom complex have deficiencies of their surface polysaccharide. We do believe that epithelial leaks are currently the most attractive theory to explain this syndrome. We do not, at this time, know what induces these leaks. It is possible that there could be defective tight junctions, poor vascular nutrients supplied to the mucosa, quantitative or qualitative deficiencies of glycosaminoglycans, or presence of urinary protamine-like substances inducing leaks. An important reason why we think PPS has the potential to help with this syndrome, is that it could plug leaks or detoxify noxious urinary polyamines. It would appear that this drug does have significant activity in patients with this symptom complex. Our study and one other confirm this activity (Fritjofsson et al. 1987) but in another study the authors felt that they could not demonstrate any activity of the medication (Holm-Bentzen et al. 1987). Although their data suggested the potential for drug activity, they did not appear to have enough individuals entered to truly answer the question (Holm-Bentzen et al. 1987).

While it is important to obtain new understanding and therapy for the syndrome of interstitial cystitis, it is also a fascinating disease to study. There is the possibility that one will discover important secrets of how the bladder surface and the epithelium protect the underlying muscle, not only relative to interstitial cystitis but to other diseases where the epithelium is violated, leading to problems such as cancer or true bacterial infections. The discoveries arising from therapies of interstitial cystitis may have more far-reaching implications than just helping that one disease, especially since PPS appears also to have activity in radiation cystitis (Parsons 1986) – a disease which may also have in part defective epithelium which accelerates the course of bladder damage.

The activity of pentosanpolysulfate in some patients with the disease complex suggest that this is a heterogeneous problem and that there may be classes of patients who have a disease that is polysaccharide sensitive. Perhaps in the future, these patients will provide more answers as to how the polysaccharides are active.

References

Fritjofsson Å, Fall M, Juhlin R, Persson BE, Ruutu M (1987) Treatment of ulcer and non-ulcer interstitial cystitis with sodium pentosanpolysulfate: a multicentre trial. J Urol 138:508–512

Gill WG, Jones KW, Ruggiero KJ (1982) Protective effects of heparin and other sulfated glycosaminoglycans on crystal adhesion to injured urothelium. J Urol 127:152–154

Holm-Bentzen M, Jacobsen F, Nerstrøm B et al. (1987) A prospective double-blind clinically controlled multicenter trial of sodium pentosanpolysulfate in the treatment of interstitial cystitis and related painful bladder disease. J Urol 138:503–507

Kaufman JE, Anderson K, Parsons CL (1987) Inactivation of anti-adherence effect of the bladder surface glycosaminoglycans as a possible mechanism for carcinogenesis. Urology 30:255–258

Parsons CL (1982) Prevention of urinary tract infection by the exogenous glycosaminoglycan sodium pentosanpolysulfate. J Urol 127:167–169

Parsons CL (1986) Successful management of radiation cystitis with sodium pentosanpolysulfate. J Urol 136:813–814

Parsons CL, Greenspan C, Mulholland SG (1975) The primary antibacterial defense mechanism of the bladder. Invest Urol 13:72–76

Parsons CL, Greenspan C, Moore SW, Mulholland SG (1977) Role of surface mucin in primary antibacterial defense of bladder. Urology 9:48–52

Parsons CL, Pollen J, Anwar H, Stauffer C, Schmidt J (1980a) Antibacterial activity of bladder surface mucin duplicated in the rabbit bladder by exogenous glycosaminoglycan (sodium pentosanpolysulfate). Infect Immun 27:876–881

Parsons CL, Stauffer C, Schmidt JD (1980b) Bladder surface glycosaminoglycans: an efficient mechanism of environmental adaptation. Science 208:605–607

Parsons CL, Stauffer C, Schmidt JD (1981) Impairment of antibacterial effect of bladder surface mucin by protamine sulfate. J Infect Dis 144:180

Parsons CL, Schmidt JD, Pollen J (1983) Successful treatment of interstitial cystitis with sodium pentosanpolysulfate. J Urol 130:51–53

Parsons CL, Danielson B, Feldstrom B (1985) Inhibition of sodium urate crystal adherence to bladder surface by polysaccharide. J Urol 134:614–616

Parsons CL, Stauffer CW, Schmidt JD (1988) Reversible inactivation of bladder surface glycosaminoglycans antibacterial activity by protamine sulfate. Infect Immun 56:1341–1343

Parsons CL, Boychuk D, Jones S, Hurst R, Callahan H (1990) Bladder surface glycosaminglycans: an epithelia permeability barrier. Invest Urol 143:140

Chapter 18

Use of Transcutaneous Electrical Nerve Stimulation in the Management of Chronic Interstitial Cystitis

M. Fall

Electroanalgesia by transcutaneous electrical nerve stimulation (TENS) is used extensively in pain conditions of different etiology. TENS is a cheap and non-destructive method, but trials of this treatment in the relief of sensory disorders of the bladder are scant. The following is a summary of four studies. These include trials using different electrode sites: intravaginal, suprapubic or common peroneal/posterior tibial nerve electrodes.

Clinical Trials

Intravaginal Versus Suprapubic Stimulation

Intravaginal electrical stimulation (IVS) may inhibit the hyperactive bladder (Fall et al. 1977a, 1977b). TENS may eliminate pain of varying etiology. To explore the possible beneficial effect of these modalities 14 women with classic interstitial cystitis (IC) of long duration were treated with either long-term IVS or TENS (Fall et al. 1980). They were randomized to either method and a clinical and urodynamic evaluation was made after 6 months to 2 years. All patients had been treated previously using different conservative methods, such as steroids, anticholinergic agents in combination with analgesics or diathermic coagulation, and all of them had been on hydrostatic bladder distension before the initiation of the trial, but with only limited palliation. The device for long-term intravaginal stimulation was a flexible electrode carrier that had been made inflatable to secure it in the proper position within the vagina. Inflation was performed in order to keep the electrodes in positions found to be individually optimal (Erlandson et al. 1977). In the case of IVS an alternating pulse of 10 Hz and a pulse width of 2 ms was used. The voltage was adjusted by the patient herself to a level at which she clearly perceived stimulation. The patient was told to wear the appliance during the day-time and to remove it at night. TENS was administered by a commercially available unit giving biphasic,

50 Hz, 0.2 ms pulses via carbon rubber electrodes, positioned suprapubically 10–15 cm apart. The effect of TENS remains for some time after stimulation is switched off and patients were therefore instructed to use the device for 2 hours twice daily, at the maximum tolerable intensity. The initial allocation of patients was done randomly, with a possible change of method if the first one failed to work, but only 5 of 7 patients completed the treatment with IVS. The major drawback of IVS was that patients had problems tolerating the intravaginal device because of pain and hypersensitivity to pressure. This problem is especially significant since several months of treatment are required to obtain a symptomatic effect. Two out of 5 patients were free from bladder pain in everyday life after IVS and voiding frequency decreased considerably. Because of a subsequent change of method the TENS group finally consisted of 9 patients. Eight of them were free from pain and noted a concomitant decrease in voiding frequency.

In 7 of 14 patients the bladder capacity during anesthesia increased. Only one patient continued IVS for a very long time: this woman had the uncommon combination of IC and detrusor instability. All but one patient on TENS continued long-term treatment. Generally, suprapubic stimulation was better tolerated and was more readily accepted. IVS is a method to be reserved for cases with concomitant bladder hyperactivity.

Long-term Follow-up of Suprapubic Stimulation

The long-term results of TENS were assessed in a series of 23 patients treated with suprapubic electrodes and high, i.e. 50 Hz, or low, i.e. 2–10 Hz, frequency stimulation (Fall 1985). All patients had stable classic interstitial cystitis. The effect on symptoms and objective findings was gradual. As a rule, pain reduction was noted 2–3 weeks after the start of TENS and the full effect was obtained after several months to more than one year of treatment. Eighteen patients were relieved from pain and urinary frequency was significantly reduced. In 13 of these 18 patients the effect of treatment was somewhat variable, however, and intervals of increased symptoms occurred. One elderly woman was unable to continue TENS because it triggered cardiac arrhythmia and she had to give up the treatment, despite symptom relief. In 4 of the 18 women an excellent result was noted. Bladder pain disappeared, voiding frequency was normalized and the bladder capacity with the patient under anesthesia was significantly increased in 3 of these 4 women. An even more remarkable finding was that lesions that had been present during repeated examinations for 13 to 23 years had disappeared completely in 2 patients and were almost invisible, and did not bleed at distension in the other 2. In 5 patients the effect of TENS was poor.

Suprapubic Stimulation in Classic and Non-Ulcer IC

Chronic interstitial cystitis is not a well-defined entity but is instead a heterogeneous group of diseases (Fall et al. 1987). In a further follow-up the results of TENS in patients with classic IC and non-ulcer disease were compared (Fall 1987). The follow-up included 20 patients with classic IC and 15 with non-ulcer IC. The results were excellent or good in 16 of the 20 patients with the classic disease and 2 of the 15 with non-ulcer disease, respectively, and symptom relief was poor in 4 of the 20 with classic and 13 of the 15 with non-ulcer IC. Patients with the classic syndrome are better candidates for TENS. The apparent curative effect in a few patients with the classic syndrome is interesting. Spontaneous healing of the stable classic IC is very rare. There are characteristic histopathologic changes in the bladder wall of patients with this condition. The disappearance of lesions should indicate a reduction in the inflammatory infiltrates and may be an example of links between the central nervous system and the immune cell system. In this context it should be noted that mucosal mast cells may be innervated under certain conditions (Newsom et al. 1983). Non-ulcer patients appear to represent a disease of different etiology or pathogenesis and do not respond very well to suprapubic stimulation.

Common Peroneal or Posterior Tibial Nerve Stimulation

McGuire et al. (1983) used a device in urinary urgency syndromes with an anal electrode combined with an electrode on the posterior tibial nerve. Subsequent trials with a positive electrode positioned transcutaneously to the common peroneal or posterior tibial nerve with a ground electrode placed on the contralateral corresponding nerves was equally successful in urinary urgency. This device was designed to treat detrusor instability, but it was also applied in 5 patients with interstitial cystitis. The philosophy of choosing posterior tibial nerve and common peroneal nerve stimulation was to utilize the old Chinese acupuncture points for the inhibition of bladder activity. It should be noted that these nerves originate in the sacral region. Stimulation at 2–10 Hz and a pulse width of 5–20 ms was used, with intensities of 5–8 V producing a low current $(50 - 100 \ \mu A)$. Four of the 5 patients improved. The continued use of this method is successful, with the disappearance of bladder lesions being noted occasionally (McGuire, personal communication).

Comment

Electrical stimulation in the treatment of interstitial cystitis is an unexplored area. So far, promising results have been seen in a small number of patients. TENS is hampered by the fact that a very long period of treatment is needed to obtain a symptomatic effect. If there is an alternative with good efficacy that is fast and simple for the patient, like transurethral resection, this would be preferred by most patients. On the other hand, electrical stimulation is a non-destructive and harmless therapy that should be tried before therapy involving risks and side-effects.

The proposed mode of action of TENS (Fig. 18.1) should be the inhibition of pain by the gate control mechanism (Melzach and Wall 1965). A direct effect on the autonomous nerve supply to the bladder has also been demonstrated (Fall et al. 1980). In animal experiments of pelvic floor stimulation this response was partly mediated through the inhibition of bladder efferents (Lindström et al. 1984). Low frequency stimulation induces a number of autonomous effects and

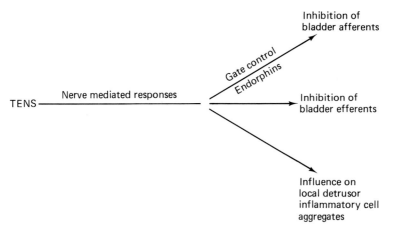

Fig. 18.1. Proposed mode of action of TENS in interstitial cystitis.

also results in the release of opiates of the central nervous system, especially endorphins (Goldstein 1976; Snyder 1977). This effect has been shown to be responsible for a decrease in the blood pressure of hypertensive rats at low frequency stimulation of the sciatic nerve for example (Yao et al. 1982).

Abortive detrusor contractions and a change in the pressure slope at cystometry is not part of the urodynamic pattern in IC. This condition is characterized by signs of a serious involvement of the sensory nerve supply to the bladder. Thus, if the effect of TENS is a result of a change in nerve activity, it is probably not mediated through an inhibition of the pelvic nerves but rather an activation of the hypogastric nerves (as registered during IVS) (Lindström et al. 1983). In this context it should be noted that different sites of stimulation, e.g. the sciatic nerves, can be used to influence the sympathetic nerve supply to the bladder (de Groat and Theobald 1976). Other possible mechanisms of TENS are the effect on hormones, mast cells or other elements. The disappearance of bladder lesions in some cases of classic IC suggests the activation of a link between the CNS and the immune cell system.

The extent of placebo effect is so far unexplored. It is difficult to design a double-blind study which is needed to clarify this issue. Treatment is based on stimulation producing a very strong sensation and no placebo equivalent of TENS is available. It has been proposed that under different pain conditions the placebo effect accounts for up to 35% of the pain reduction during treatments (Beecher 1960). A non-specific placebo effect of this magnitude may thus also exist with TENS.

The results of TENS could possibly be further improved. The optimal site of stimulation is so far unknown. Suprapubic stimulation involves thoracolumbar segments and common peroneal and tibial nerve stimulation involves the sacral segments. This could result in different effects and should be further evaluated. Other sites for stimulation should be explored. The choice of stimulation parameters should also be further investigated. High frequency stimulation elicits effects different from those of acupuncture type low frequency stimulation, which can essentially be regarded as a muscle stimulation. The patients treated with suprapubic stimulation whose bladder lesions healed all had high frequency stimulation for a very long time. On the other hand, pain relief seems to be faster when low frequency stimulation is used. So far, most of the available data are preliminary and further studies are needed to determine the usefulness and mechanisms of action of electrical stimulation in interstitial cystitis.

References

Beecher HK (1960) Increased stress and effectiveness of placebo and "active" drugs. Science 132:91–92

de Groat WC, Theobald RJ (1976) Reflex activation of sympathetic pathways to vesical smooth muscle and parasympathetic ganglia by electrical stimulation of vesical afferents. J Physiol 259:223–237

Erlandson BE, Fall M, Sundin T (1977) Intravaginal electrical stimulation. Clinical experiments on urethral closure. Scand J Urol Nephrol [Suppl] 44:31–40

Fall M (1985) Conservative management of chronic interstitial cystitis: transcutaneous electrical nerve stimulation and transurethral resection. J Urol 133:774–778

Fall M (1987) Transcutaneous electrical nerve stimulation in interstitial cystitis: up-date on clinical experience. Urology 24 [Suppl]:40–42

Fall M, Erlandson BE, Carlsson C-A, Lindström S (1977a) The effect of intravaginal electrical stimulation on the feline urethra and urinary bladder. Scand J Urol Nephrol [Suppl] 44:19–30.

Fall M, Erlandson BE, Sundin T, Waagstien F (1977b) Intravaginal electrical stimulation. Clinical experiments on bladder inhibition. Scand J Urol Nephrol [Suppl] 44:41–47

Fall M, Carlsson C-A, Erlandson BE (1980) Electrical stimulation in interstitial cystitis. J Urol 123:192–195

Fall M, Johansson SL, Aldenborg F (1987) Chronic interstitial cystitis: a heterogeneous syndrome. J Urol 137:35–38

Goldstein A (1976) Opioid peptides (endorphins) in pituitary and brain. Science 193:1081–1086

Lindström S, Fall M, Carlsson CA, Erlandson BE (1983) The neurophysiological basis of bladder inhibition in response to intravaginal electrical stimulation. J Urol 129:405–410

Lindström S, Fall M, Carlsson C-A, Erlandson BE (1984) Rhythmic activity in pelvic efferents to the bladder: an experimental study in the cat with reference to the clinical condition "unstable bladder". Urol Int 39:272–279

McGuire EJ, Shi-Chun Z, Horwinski ER, Lytton B (1983) Treatment of motor and sensory detrusor instability by electrical stimulation. J Urol 129:78–79

Melzach R, Wall PD (1965) Pain mechanisms: a new theory. Science 150:971–979

Newson B, Dahlström A, Enerbäck L, Ahlman H (1983) Suggestive evidence for a direct innervation of mucosal mast cells. An electron microscopic study. Neuroscience 10:565–570

Snyder SH (1977) Opiate receptors in the brain. N Engl J Med 296:266–271

Yao T, Andersson S, Thorén P (1982) Long-lasting cardiovascular depressor response following sciatic stimulation in spontaneously hypertensive rat. Evidence for the involvement of central endorphin and serotonin systems. Brain Res 244:295–303.

Chapter 19

Reappraisal of Transurethral Resection in Classic Interstitial Cystitis

M. Fall

Introduction

The resection of bladder wall lesions had been found to diminish symptoms in interstitial cystitis (Hunner 1918, Frankson 1957). Since lesions are usually multiple, open resection is difficult and even inappropriate in most patients. Kerr (1971) was the first to describe the successful treatment of interstitial cystitis by transurethral resection (TUR) as a case report. Greenberg and associates (1974) used the method systematically in 28 patients with irritative voiding, urinary frequency and suprapubic pain and tenderness. All patients had a typical lesion of the Hunner type and all of them had a diminished bladder capacity of 210 ml or less. Only patients who failed on various types of non-surgical therapy or had very severe symptoms and cystoscopic findings were chosen for TUR. Resection included the bladder mucosa and submucosa but not the bladder muscle. All patients improved for varying periods of time. In 3 recurrence was noted within less than 1 year, in 17 symptomatic recurrence occurred between 1 and 3 years after TUR, 1 improved for more than 3 years and in 4 patients no recurrence was noted during follow-up. When there was a recurrence the treatment was repeated. Greenberg also tried transurethral fulguration in 7 cases. In 5 there was some improvement, but recurrence occurred within less than 1 year and in 2 no improvement was obtained.

This mode of treatment was discontinued after only 7 cases because of disappointing results. In a recently published series systematic TUR was also found to produce a good palliative effect in interstitial cystitis (Fall 1985). Thirty patients were treated with a complete TUR of visible lesions. All macroscopically affected areas were resected including the mucosa, submucosa and half or more of the muscular coat. The initial effect was excellent in 11 patients with the disappearance of pain and normalization of urinary frequency. In a further 10 patients the pain disappeared and urinary frequency was reduced significantly. Nine were free of pain but had persistent urinary frequency. The duration of symptom palliation ranged from 2 to 42 months. All patients had been on distension therapy before resection. A comparison of the symptomatic improvement after distension and TUR showed a very marked difference, with only a short effect for distension.

The removal of local changes in the bladder wall, which is thought to be more or less generally involved in the disease, has been looked upon with scepticism by many urologists. There is, however, no doubt that within the circumscript lesions of classic interstitial cystitis the histopathologic changes (e.g. perineural and perivascular lymphocyte and plasma cell infiltrations and the increased number of mast cells) are more prominent than in cystoscopically normal areas (Smith and Dehner 1972; Fall et al. 1985; Aldenborg et al. 1986). The removal of these areas may influence the course of the disease. The following is an update on the experience of TUR of classic interstitial cystitis.

Update on the Author's Own Experience

Forty-six women and 3 men aged between 25 and 84 years (mean age 62 years) were treated. The duration of symptoms ranged from 1 to 30 years. All patients had the characteristic pain on bladder filling, which was relieved partly or completely by voiding. They also suffered from moderate to very marked urinary frequency. All patients in the present series had the classic signs at cystoscopy with anesthesia; single (6 patients) or multiple mucosal areas with small radiating vessels converging in a central small coagulum, fibrin deposit (Fig. 19.1) or scar, which ruptured during distension of the bladder (Fig. 19.2), with petechial oozing of blood from the ulcer bottom and the mucosal margins. After distension a mild bullous swelling was observed in the periphery of the lesion (Fig. 19.3). This area was also resected. At the primary investigation glomerulations were seen, although these varied in number.

In all patients bladder capacity was determined during anesthesia at a pressure of 70 cm of water, with the identification of bladder lesions. A low-pressure continuous irrigation resectoscope was used to permit continuous resection with a constant volume within the bladder. All lesions were carefully identified for complete resection and all involved areas were removed with the diathermia equipment preset at pure cutting at as low an intensity as possible. The resection included half or more of the muscular coat underlying the lesions. Direct pin-point coagulation of bleeding vessels was performed and fulguration of the resected surfaces was avoided. An indwelling catheter was left in situ postoperatively until the urine became clear. The effect of the treatment was assessed from the patients' reports of bladder pain. They also kept voiding charts covering 48 hour periods, every month to begin with, and every 6 months in the case of stable improvement. Cystoscopy with the registration of bladder capacity and monitoring of the bladder lesions was performed every 6–12 months.

There was an initial decrease of pain in all patients. In 5, however, the pain did not completely disappear. Urinary frequency also decreased initially. In 18 patients the pain was abolished after only one resection and the good effect has so far lasted from 1 up to 7 years, mean 3 years (Table 19.1). In 11 patients there has been a long-lasting abolition of pain after a second TUR, with a duration of 0.5 to 5 years (mean 3 years). In 12 patients two or three TURs have not resulted in long-lasting pain relief. Seven of them have required TUR once or twice a

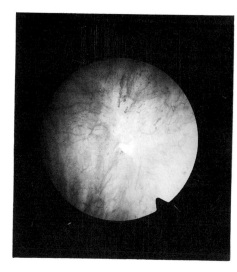

Fig. 19.1. Bladder mucosa during initial phase of blader distension. Small radiating vessels converging in a pale central scar with fibrin deposit.

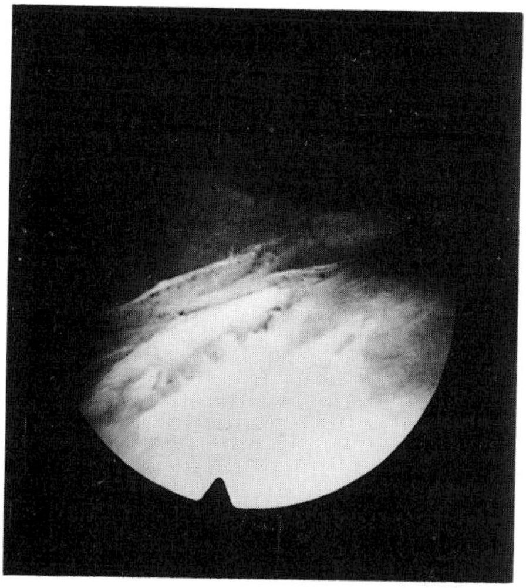

Fig. 19.2. Rupture of bladder mucosa and submucosa at increased bladder distension.

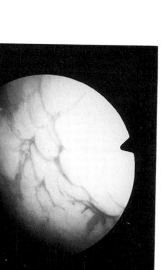

Fig. 19.3. Mild bullous swelling and reddening of the mucosa at periphery of bladder lesion after distension.

Table 19.1. Number of therapeutic TURs in 49
patients

1	in 18 patients lasting effect
2	in 11 patients lasting effect
3–4	in 3 patients lasting effect
>2	in 12 patients no lasting effect
1	in 5 patients follow-up too short

year to stay acceptably free from symptoms and for them other methods have
been instituted. One woman has had six TURs in 8 years with a satisfactory
effect each time and she refuses other forms of therapy. In 4 patients TUR was
abandoned because of severe urinary frequency and progressive bladder
contracture. In 5 patients there is no adequate follow-up.

The recurrence of urinary frequency usually occurred before the recurrence of
pain. The majority of patients, also the subjects with persistent pain relief, had
urinary frequency. In the long-term perspective this component was not as
effectively controlled as bladder pain. However, although frequency was evident
from their micturition charts, few patients complained. Most of them were

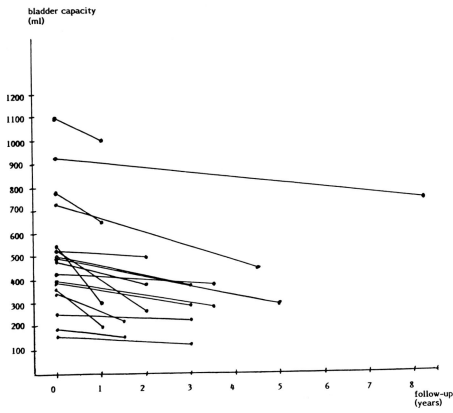

Fig. 19.4. Degree of decrease of bladder capacity during follow-up in 18 patients treated by TUR.

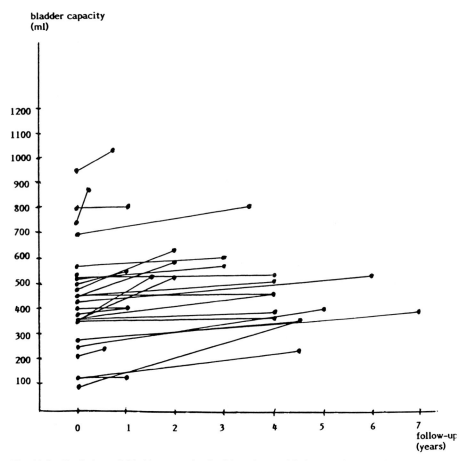

Fig. 19.5. Evolution of bladder capacity in 26 patients with increased or unchanged capacity following TUR.

satisfied as long as pain control was adequate and urinary frequency not too extreme.

Repeated TURs were necessary to control the symptoms in the majority of patients. Except for cases requiring yearly resections, the time interval between the second and third resection generally increased compared to the interval between the first and second one. At cystoscopy the bladder mucosa had a less irritated appearance after healing of the TUR: less prominent vascular injection, no reddening of the mucosa, less pronounced mucosal edema after distension and few petechial bleedings. The endoscopic feature looked less "active". Prominent scarring of the bladder wall at the site of resection was a rule rather than an exception. This finding was, however, nor correlated to decreased bladder capacity during anesthesia. Eighteen of 49 patients demonstrated a moderate to marked decrease of capacity, while 26 had an increased or unchanged capacity during anesthesia (Figs 19.4 and 19.5). In 5 patients so far no follow-up measurement of bladder capacity has been possible. The immediate complications of TUR were few and easily handled: extraperitoneal bladder perforations in 5 patients and prolonged bleeding after seven resections, complications treated with prolonged catheter drainage lasting between 2 and 5 days.

Comments

The object of transurethral resection is to remove the most affected areas of the bladder. This does not result in the eradication of the disease. On the contrary, symptomatic recurrence is to be expected sooner or later. The endoscopic changes do not disappear, but as a rule the endoscopic signs of inflammation decrease. A more or less prominent post-resection scar develops with a reduced number of radiating vessels, few post-distension glomerulations and little post-distension edema. The fragility of the mucosa persists with the central rupture of scars during distension. Resection should be performed at low intensity and without general fulguration so as not to increase scarring more than necessary. Fulguration alone is inefficient and seems to be a hazardous procedure in interstitial cystitis since it probably enhances the scar formation. The strong tendency to scar formation in this disease may be a result of the mast cell promotion of fibroblasts. TUR results in the removal of areas with maximum mast cell involvement.

To what extent can increased scarring be related to transurethral resection, with a possible development towards bladder contracture? This question can only be answered by repeated, reliable measurement of bladder capacity. To be able to determine whether capacity during anesthesia has changed, measurement has to be performed in a very strict manner. The patient should be kept under deep general or spinal/epidural anesthesia. Infusion should go on until no more fluid escapes into the bladder and the superimposed intravesical pressure should be constant at every measurement (e.g. 70 cm of water). The urethra should be obstructed by compression if leakage occurs around the cystoscope. Several consecutive measurements on different occasions are required to determine the trend of capacity change. In one-third of the present cases a decreased capacity was noted, while registered bladder volume increased or was essentially unchanged in the majority of patients. Thus, resections seem to result in local scars rather than general scarring of the detrusor. It should be remembered that bladder contracture occurs as part of the natural course of interstitial cystitis. It was noted that patients with an aggressive, general reaction of the bladder mucosa seemed to develop bladder contracture rather quickly. In the present series no clear indications were found suggesting that TUR enhances this process.

There can be arguments about the mechanisms of the beneficial effect of TUR. This study was an open one with each patient serving as his/her own control. The therapeutic effect cannot be due to prolonged bladder distension: since an irrigative cystoscope was used there was no prolonged, high-pressure overdistension. The effect of a standard 10-minute overdistension at 70 cm of water has been compared with TUR. The effect of distension was much more short-lived (Fall 1985). Generally it can be assumed that a placebo effect would disappear quickly in patients with classic interstitial cystitis, a well-defined

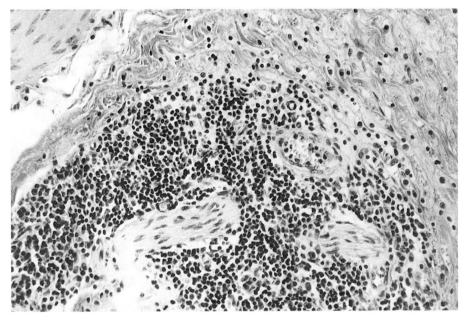

Fig. 19.6. Dense perineural infiltrate of lymphocytes and plasma cells in resected lesion of patient with classic interstitial cystitis.

disease of long duration in patients who have been subjected to multiple therapeutic trials for many years. The placebo effect is perhaps more marked in patients with non-ulcer interstitial cystitis (Fritjofsson et al. 1987).

The control of pain by TUR was substantial in this series. In many cases this essential effect had a very long duration. The effect on urinary frequency was more variable and less durable. What is the explanation of symptom relief after TUR? The local resection of intramural nerves and the removal of inflammatory cell aggregates, which influence local innervation, are possible explanations (Fig. 19.6). TUR can be looked upon as a very peripheral denervation. The less pronounced effect on frequency shows that the disease is not eradicated: instead TUR puts the disease into remission, either partly or completely. Resections of single lesions were associated with an exceptionally good prognosis, while resections in patients with a pronounced general reaction were unsuccessful in the long term. It follows that good clinical experience with the cystoscopic findings, as well as the ability to evaluate the extent of the lesions and also to perform a complete resection, is important.

References

Aldenborg F, Fall M, Enerbäck L (1986) Proliferation and transepithelial migration of mucosal mast cells in interstitial cystitis. Immunology 58:411–416

Fall M (1985) Conservative management of chronic interstitial cystitis: transcutaneous electrical nerve stimulation and transurethral resection. J Urol 133:774–778

Fall M, Johansson SL, Vahlne A (1985) A clinicopathological and virological study of interstitial cystitis. J Urol 133:771–773

Frankson C (1957) Interstitial cystitis: a clinical study of 59 cases. Acta Chir Scand 113:51–62

Fritjofsson A, Fall M. Juhlin R, Persson BE, Ruutu M (1987) Treatment of ulcer and non-ulcer interstitial cystitis with sodium pentosanpolysulfate (Elmiron): a multicenter trial. J Urol 138:508–512

Greenberg E, Barnes R, Stewart S, Furnish T (1974) Transurethral resection of Hunner's ulcer. J Urol 111:764–766

Hunner GL (1918) Elusive ulcer of the bladder: further notes on a rare type of bladder ulcer with report of 25 cases. Am J Obstet 78:374–395

Kerr Jr WS (1971) Interstitial cystitis: treatment by transurethral resection. J Urol 105:664–666

Smith BH, Dehner LP (1972) Chronic ulcerating interstitial cystitis (Hunner's ulcer). A study of 28 cases. Arch Pathol 93:77–81

Chapter 20

Treatment of Interstitial Cystitis with the Neodymium: YAG Laser

A.M. Shanberg and T. Malloy

The use of the neodymium:yttrium aluminum garnet (Nd:YAG) laser in the treatment of superficial carcinoma of the bladder was first described by Staehler and Hofstetter in the 1970s. Since that time, other authors have confirmed the usefulness of this new modality of therapy in the treatment of both superficial and invasive carcinoma of the bladder (Smith 1986; Beisland et al. 1985). The methodology used is to photoirradiate the bladder carcinoma with the Nd:YAG laser, delivered via a fiberoptic bundle passed through a cystoscope, until the bladder wall and tumor turn a chalk-white in appearance. This visual end point has been shown to correspond to heating the protein in the cells of the bladder to approximately 60–70°C. At this temperature the elastic fibers of the bladder are not damaged (Hofstetter and Frank 1980). Over the next 4–6 weeks the cells of the tumor and bladder wall necrose, slough off, and are replaced with healthy collagen fibers. If too high a laser energy is used, the tissue vaporizes or turns black with superficial carbonization, which is a process to be discouraged because of the increased absorption of laser energy superficially by the carbonization itself.

In the treatment of the bladder wall in patients with interstitial cystitis, we have found it necessary to lower the wattage of energy used to prevent the phenomenon of forward scatter of the laser beam, which could damage structures adjacent to the bladder. Forward scatter means that anything up to 20% of the laser energy focused on the bladder can pass through the bladder wall (without burning a hole through the bladder) and be absorbed by small or large intestine contiguous with the bladder. This may then result in necrosis of bowel wall with subsequent perforation of either small or large intestine in, generally 48–72 hours after laser therapy.

The possible causes of interstitial cystitis have been covered in detail elsewhere in this book. Our criteria for diagnosis of interstitial cystitis were that all our patients had to have deep bladder biopsies performed confirming the presence of inflammatory cells in the submucosal areas of the bladder and/or the lamina propria and muscle layers of the bladder (Fig. 20.1A). All patients also had bladder cytology to exclude carcinoma in situ and intravenous pyelograms to rule out other associated urologic disease. In patients with an associated

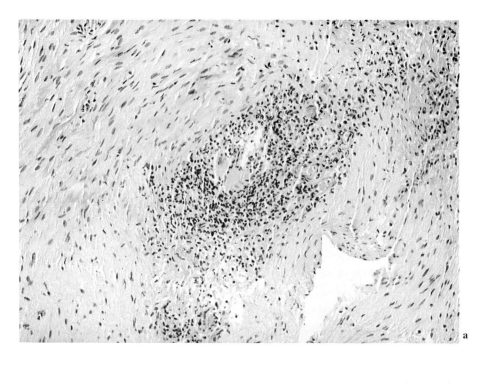

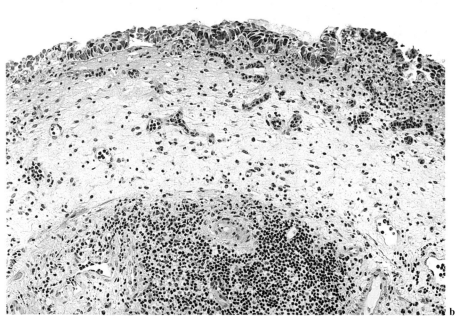

Fig. 20.1. a Microscopic biopsy of interstitial cystitis. **b** Microscopic ulceration from interstitial cystitis.

Hunner's ulcer disease, the biopsy not only showed the typical inflammatory changes, but also the endothelial layer of the bladder was consistent with ulceration. (Fig. 20.1B).

Attempts were made to measure mast cell infiltrate and increased numbers of mast cells, but in our patients there was no significant increase in mast cell infiltrate compared with biopsies performed for other reasons in other patients. All patients without the inflammatory changes described above were eliminated from this study.

The use of the resectoscope to treat Hunner's ulcer disease was originally reported by Greenberg et al. (1974), with a fairly good palliative response. In another group of patients with Hunner's ulcers associated with interstitial cystitis, Fall (1985) used a combination of transurethral resection and transcutaneous electrical nerve stimulation to treat this disease. He claimed that complete transurethral resection resulted in the disappearance of pain in all of his 30 patients and a decrease in frequency in 21 of those patients that he evaluated.

We have felt that a possible problem with the use of transurethral resection with an electrocautery is the chronic scarring effect seen in patients with multiple resections for bladder tumors. Hypothetically this can result in further decreased bladder capacity in this group of patients. The Nd:YAG laser has been used by ourselves and others in the treatment of patients with bladder carcinoma (Shanberg et al. 1987) and we have not observed any decrease in bladder capacity despite multiple treatments in patients since 1982. As we shall discuss later, the laser only rarely cures this disease, usually only palliating the symptomatology; consequently retreatments frequently become necessary.

Materials and Methods

Since our intital report in 1985 (IDEM 1985), 39 patients who have fulfilled the preceding criteria have been treated at two institutions in the following manner. The bladder, under anesthesia, is first distended to vizualize any petechial hemorrhages or ulcer craters (Fig. 20.2a,b). The bladder is then collapsed and treated in the collapsed state by photoirradiating the ulcerated area and a surrounding 1 cm area of normal bladder wall. The markedly inflamed areas are also photoirradiated until the bladder wall turns chalk white (Fig. 20.2c), to correspond to heating the tissue to 60–70°C. The laser is set to 25–30 watts and a 3 second pulse duration, the fiberoptic tip being placed 1–3 mm from the bladder wall using a spot size of 2–3 mm. If the ureteral orifices are involved, they are also photoirradiated in a similar manner. The patient is kept in an extreme Trendelenburg position, and the fiberoptic tip is kept in constant motion to attempt to decrease the risk of small-bowel perforation.

The total dosage (watts × seconds = joules) of laser energy is restricted to 25 000 joules at one session in each patient. Some of our patients have had to be retreated more than once because of extensive disease and the limitation recently placed on total dosage.

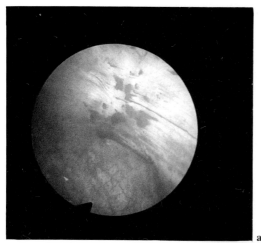

a

Fig. 20.2. a Endoscopic view: petechial
hemorrhage with interstitial cystitis.
b Hunner's ulcer with interstitial cystitis.
c Laser treated bladder with interstitial
cystitis.

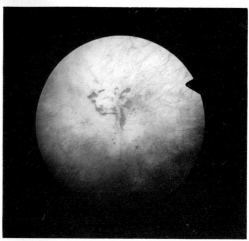

b

c

Results and Conclusions

Thirty-three females and 6 males were treated. Their age range is shown in Fig. 20.3. All patients in this series have had prior treatment and have been failures of prior treatment regimens – usually DMSO bladder instillations, but also including silver nitrate instillations, hydraulic stretching of the bladder, and oxychlorosene sodium bladder instillations. All patients were admitted to the hospital for at least one night's observation, and the majority were discharged after hospitalization of one or two nights.

There were 19 patients with Hunner's ulcer disease who had biopsies. Of these 19 patients, 17 reported rapid relief of pain generally in the first week after treatment, occasionally not until 4–6 weeks post-treatment; 1 patient reported mild improvement, but refused further therapy; and 1 patient had no benefit from photoirradiation. Twelve of the 17 patients with a good result reported recurrence of symptoms between 6 and 18 months post-treatment; 9 were retreated and 3 were managed successfully with DMSO and anticholinergic drug therapy. Bladder capacity increased by more than 100 ml, and nocturia was decreased in 14 of the 17 patients. Two of the remaining 3 patients required augmentation cystoplasty for a markedly decreased bladder capacity, but their pain never recurred after laser therapy.

The remaining 20 patients without Hunner's ulcer disease but with biopsy-proven interstitial cystitis, were also evaluated in terms of decreased pain, decreased frequency, and improvement in bladder capacity (greater than 100 ml). Of these 20 patients, 13 felt they had marked improvement of symptoms and objective evidence of increased bladder capacity (65%); 3 had

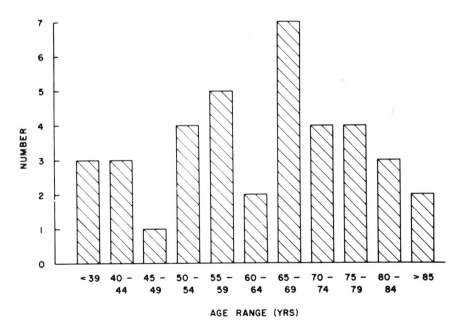

Fig. 20.3.   Age range of patients with interstitial cystitis.

temporary improvement for several months, then symptoms recurred, but they refused further therapy (15%); and 4 had no improvement and were considered failures (20%).

In 2 patients in this overall series of 39 patients, small-bowel perforations developed several days after laser photoirradiation therapy. This occurred prior to the dosimetry being restricted to 25 watts of energy and a total of 25 000 joules. Since that time we have not seen any small-bowel perforations.

In summary, the majority of our patients with biopsy-proven interstitial cystitis and Hunner's ulcer disease showed an improvement of their symptoms after Nd:YAG laser photoirradiation therapy (17 of 19), especially relief of the severe pain associated with this disease. Many of these patients have required retreatment, since the disease develops in other areas of the bladder not photoirradiated, anywhere from 6–18 months after initial treatment. Patients without Hunner's ulcers but with pain have also shown improvement (65%), but not as dramatic a response as was seen in those with ulcers.

The laser, because of its unique effect of causing a full thickness (2–3 mm) destruction of the inflamed bladder wall without damage to the elastic fibers in the bladder, has resulted in an improvement of the bladder capacity and symptoms in this group of patients.

Nd:YAG laser photoirradiation definitely is not a permanent cure for this disease of unknown etiology, but can offer palliation to a large percentage of patients with biopsy-proven evidence of interstitial cystitis. This is a critical criterion for treatment, as obviously many inflammatory states of the bladder can mimic interstitial cystitis and in our experience when several of these patients were treated there was absolutely no benefit from photoirradiation therapy.

References

Beisland HO, Sander S, Fossberg E (1985) Neodymium:YAG laser irradiation of urinary bladder tumor. Follow-up study of 100 consecutively treated patients. Urol 25:559

Fall M (1985) Conservative management of chronic interstitial cystitis transcutaneous electrical nerve stimulation and transurethral resection. J Urol 133:744

Greenberg E, Barnes R, Stewart S, Furnish T (1974) Transurethral resection of Hunner's ulcer. J Urol 111:764

Hofstetter A, Frank F (1980) The neodymium-YAG laser in urology. Hoffman-La Roche and Co, Basel

IDEM (1985) Treatment of interstitial cystitis with the neodymium-YAG laser, J Urol 134:885

Shanberg A, Baghdassarian R, Tansey L (1987) Use of the Nd:YAG laser in the treatment of bladder cancer. Urology 29:26

Smith JA (1986) Treatment of invasive bladder carcinoma with a Neodymium:YAG laser. J Urol 135:55

Staehler GW, Hofstetter A (1979) A transurethral laser irradiation of urinary bladder tumors. Eur Urol 5:64

Chapter 21

Partial Bladder Denervation in the Treatment of Interstitial Cystitis in Women

A. Ingelman-Sundberg

Introduction

Denervation in cases of interstitial cystitis has been performed in various ways. Extended resections of the external layers of bladder wall have been attempted. Overdistension of the bladder can at least temporarily defunctionalize the nerves in the bladder wall, and a temporary effect can be achieved by transurethral injections of phenol solutions beneath the bladder base.

Resection of sacral nerve roots has also been accomplished. During this operation it may be difficult to avoid damage to nerves regulating the rectal function even if microdissection is used. A much simpler method is to resect the nerves in the lower part of the parametrium corrsponding to the inferior hypogastric plexus (Ingelman-Sundberg 1959). During the resection in this region both sympathetic and parasympathetic nerves to the bladder are cut, whereas the nerves to other pelvic organs are left intact.

Indications

The method is recommended for selected cases after conventional treatment has failed. Patient selection is made by application of local anesthesia in both parametria. The test is carried out as follows.

Selection of Patients

Twenty millilitres of a solution containing 5 mg lidocaine and 5 μg adrenaline per ml is injected into the anterior fornix on both sides 1 cm lateral to the cervix and at a depth of about 3 cm (Fig. 21.1). Urethrocystometry curves are recorded before the injection and 5 minutes after it has been finished. The patient is then

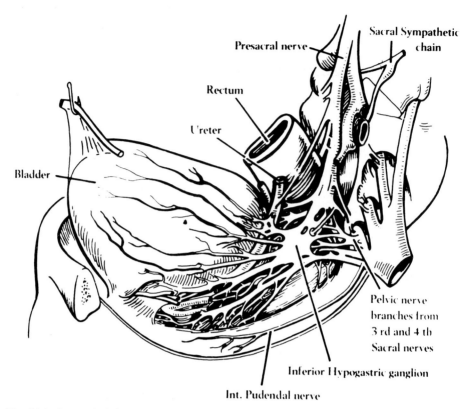

Fig. 21.1. Anatomical drawing showing the lateral aspect of the left inferior hypogastric plexus. Local anesthesia is applied corresponding to the site of the inferior hypogastric ganglion.

allowed to walk around to test the effect of the anesthesia herself. When she cannot hold the urine any longer she is allowed to micturate. The urine volume is measured as well as the amount of residual urine. If the residual urine is more than 150 ml only unilateral resection is recommended. If the urgency and the bladder capacity are unaffected by the anesthesia there is no indication for surgery.

Operative Technique

The patient is placed in the lithotomy position.

1. A transverse incision is made below the external urethral orifice and the anterior vaginal wall is dissected free up to the cervix exposing the pubocervical fascia and the pubococcygeus muscles. (Fig. 21.2).

2. A long clamp or long pair of scissors is now inserted into the tissue between the pubocervical fascia and the pubococcygeus muscle and opened.

3. Long retractors are introduced into the tissue at the same place and separated (Fig. 21.3). The inferior hypogastric plexus is then often immediately exposed appearing lateral to the rectum and following the inferior vesical

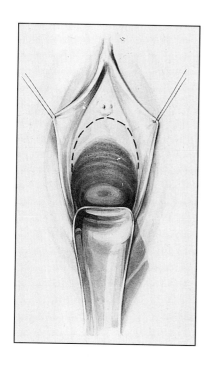

Fig. 21.2. Transverse incision below the external urethral orifice.

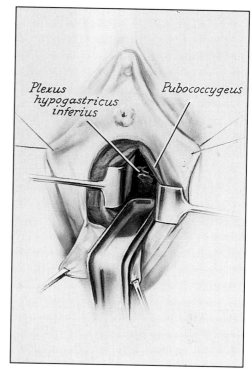

Fig. 21.3. Exposure of the inferior hypogastric plexus.

vessels. If necessary further dissection is performed by using two long dissecting forceps.

4. When the nerves are laid free, they are grasped between two long clamps and resected. Often the nerve fibers are difficult to isolate from the vessels. the nerves and the vessels can then be resected at the same time. A diathermy electrode is put on the clamps and the tissue grasped in them is electrocoagulated after a check has been made that the ureter is at a safe distance from the clamps.

5. If the operation is to be bilateral the corresponding steps are carried out on the other side.

6. The vaginal wall is reapproximated and sutured.

7. A suprapubic catheter is introduced and the vagina is packed for 24 hours.

Post-Operative Management

Bladder training by clamping and releasing the catheter 2–4 hourly is started immediately, and the catheter can usually be removed after 1–2 days. The patient is allowed to get out of bed 1 hour after packing has been removed. She is instructed to measure the volume of urine when urinating and to note the result.

Results

The method has been used in 10 cases, all with a typical anamnesis and a Hunner's ulcer. In 3 the anesthesia had no effect on the bladder capacity, probably because there was already too much fibrosis in the bladder wall. No operation was therefore performed. In 7 cases the effect was good and a bilateral nerve resection was made. Two patients were cured and 5 much improved. The time of observation is now 5 years or more. In Fig. 21.4 a typical case is illustrated.

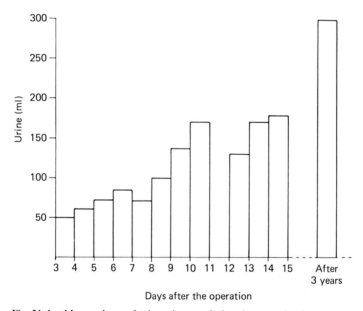

Fig. 21.4. Mean volume of urine micturated after the operation in a case of interstitial cystitis.

References

Ingelman-Sundberg A (1959) Partial denervation of the bladder. A new method for the treatment of urge incontinence and similar conditions in women. Acta Obstet Gynecol Scand 38:487–502
Ingelman-Sundberg A (1975) Urge incontinence in women. Acta Obstet Gynecol Scand 54:153–156
Obrink A, Bunne G, Ingelman-Sundberg A (1978) Urethral pressure in urge incontinence and after hypogastric blockade. Urol Int 33:107–110

Chapter 22

Surgical Therapy of Interstitial Cystitis

A. Siegel, J. Snyder and S. Raz

Introduction

Any disease process that has a multitude of therapeutic approaches is generally a condition without a truly effective treatment (Hanno and Wein 1987). Interstitial cystitis is such an entity and remains enigmatic and problematic with respect to its etiology, pathology, diagnosis and treatment. The only certainty is that it is an important lesion causing transmural inflammation of the bladder wall which confers on its victim marked irritative voiding symptoms and consequentially intense misery and suffering. According to Messing (Messing and Stamey 1978), the hallmark of interstitial cystitis is glomerulation upon the second bladder distension and the characteristic histological finding is submucosal edema and vasodilation. An infiltrate of mast cells is characteristically found in the bladder wall.

Surgical Treatment

The surgical treatment of interstitial cystitis is an absolute last resort after all trials of conservative treatment have failed; a point which cannot be over-emphasized. It must be remembered that interstitial cystitis, although causing significant morbidity, is a non-malignant process which does not cause mortality. Nowhere does the caveat "primum non nocere" bear more relevance; the treatment must be no worse than the disease process. Essentially, surgery is reserved for "bladder cripples", a term which encompasses approximately 10% of the interstitial cystitis population with severe and intractable disease (Oravisto 1975).

The gamut of surgical therapy ranges from endoscopic manipulation to surgical extirpation. Hydraulic distension, transurethral resection, fulguration, or laser therapy, neurosurgical ablative procedures, cystolysis, cysto-cystoplasty, augmentation cystoplasty with supra-trigonal cystectomy, and total cystectomy with diversion or bladder replacement have been utilized as therapeutic alternatives. According to Messing (Messing and Stamey 1978), the only certain method of achieving total symptomatic relief is supra-vesical urinary diversion, with or without cystectomy.

Bumpus (1930) first described the therapeutic effect of bladder distension in 1930. This method provides symptomatic relief in about 30% of patients (Messing 1986). Many different regimens with respect to intravesical pressure and time have been described. Irrespectively, the mechanism of treatment seems to be ischemic and/or mechanical damage to the submucosal afferent nerve plexus or stretch receptors with subsequent blunting of the pain sensation and increase in capacity (Pool 1967). Dunn et al. (1977) demonstrated that bladder distension to systolic pressure for 1.3 hours under epidural anesthesia led to tripling of bladder capacity which was sustained, but to a lesser extent, 3 to 6 months later. An unfortunate complication was bladder rupture in 8% of patients.

Transurethral resection or fulguration of discrete ulcers has resulted in favorable responses with regard to increasing bladder capacity (Fall 1985). Greenberg and colleagues (1974) reported 60% of 35 patients to be symptom-free for more than one year after treatment. Shanberg and co-workers (1985) reported encouraging results utilizing neodymium:YAG laser phototherapy with short-term follow-up. However, a survey of 25 interstitial cystitis patients who underwent laser therapy revealed only about 10% with any improvement at all, and these were the patients with the "Hunner's ulcer" type of interstitial cystitis, that is, those with discrete ulcers. The majority of patients had either no improvement at all or were worse for about a 6 week period of time, after which return to baseline status occurred (personal communication 1987). Hunner (Hunner 1918) used partial cystectomy to treat ulcers but found that this resulted in worsening of symptoms and decrease in capacity. One question that remains unanswered is does the therapeutic effect of the concomitant hydrodistension accompanying any of these endoscopic procedures account for more of the therapeutic response than the specific endoscopic manipulation? A major criticism of any procedure that treats specific focal lesions is that interstitial cystitis is a disease of a diffuse nature which requires a diffuse treatment approach.

Open neurosurgical ablative procedures including presacral neurectomy (Borque 1951), bilateral cordotomy (Hanash and Pool 1969) and differential sacral neurectomy (Lapides 1975) have been reportedly successful in anecdotal cases. Torrens (Torrens and Hald 1979) reported that bladder denervation procedures can provide bladder rehabilitation when other measures have failed. Procedures performed in proximity to the bladder are generally more successful than those in proximity to the spinal cord. These procedures average a 50% improvement although long-term follow-up remains to be seen. An important caveat is that no denervation procedure will work with a contracted bladder.

Turner-Warwick and Ashkan (1967) described a technique called cysto-cystoplasty in which the bladder is circumferentially transected and then reanastamosed, a procedure that will theoretically destroy intramural nerves and might confer increased capacity and symptomatic relief. From this procedure evolved cystolysis, a denervation procedure described by Worth and Turner-Warwick in 1973 (Worth and Turner-Warwick 1973). Most of the sensory pathways subserving the upper part of the bladder are destroyed by dividing the superior vesical pedicle and the ascending branches of the inferior vesical pedicle, leaving the bladder base, peritoneal patch, and ureters intact. Unfortunately, the results of cystolysis have been variable, with capacity under anesthesia improving in only half. Freiha and Stamey (1980) reported post-cystolysis urodynamic findings of increased capacity, acontractile detrusor, maintained sensation of distension, and voiding by Valsalva. They claimed a theoretical advantage of selective denervation without interfering with sphincteric or bladder base sensation. They claimed a success in 5–6 patients followed for up to 30 months. Leach and Raz (Leach and Raz 1983) reported 28–32 patients with partial or complete pain relief, but 6 had continued frequency and 7 failed to void. Long-term follow-up of these patients demonstrated the development of abnormal cystometry with hypertonic, poorly compliant filling curves. Many patients ultimately required augmentation cytoplasty to increase bladder capacity. Most of the patients whom on short-term follow-up were found to have pain relief ultimately redeveloped pain; only 7 patients had pain relief on long-term follow-up. The phenomenon of nerve reinnervation with sprouting of fibers is an attractive hypothesis to explain the poor results of cystolysis. In view of the fact that the bladder cannot be completely denervated and our unsatisfactory long-term results, we are no longer recommending this procedure. Similarly, Worth (1980) concluded that cystolysis yielded unpredictable long-term results.

In a similar vein, endoscopic methods have been utilized to effect denervation while avoiding a major open surgical procedure. Endoscopic supra-ureteric bladder transection via a circumferential incision (Borque 1951), endoscopic subtrigonal phenol injection (Hanash and Pool 1969), as well as supra-trigonal circumferential neodymium:YAG laser phototherapy (Shanberg, et al. 1985) have all been attempted with mixed results.

Augmentation Cystoplasty

Objectives and Goals

Ideally, the goal of surgery for interstitial cystitis is to provide complete relief, if not significant improvement, of the distressing symptoms for which the patient has sought treatment. There are six "cardinal" symptoms of interstitial cystitis for which patients seek treatment, all of which may or may not be present. These symptoms include the following:

1. Urinary frequency and urgency
2. Pain during sexual intercourse
3. Burning during urination
4. Pain during bladder filling relieved by voiding
5. Constant pelvic pain
6. Mental stress due to the severity of the above symptoms, the difficulties encountered in trying to perform normal life activities, and the resultant

depression, adjustment difficulties, and feelings of isolation from society
These problems are compounded by the fact that these patients in seeking an answer to their problem, see many physicians, are the recipients of many different treatment modalities, and often receive few answers and sustain no improvement. In fact, sometimes mental stress precedes the appearance of the physical symptoms. This brings up the question of the possibility of a neuro-humoral mechanism accounting for this phenomenon.

It is fundamental to recognize that any form of surgical therapy can address some of the symptoms, but rarely all of these symptoms. To avoid unrealistic expectations after surgery, patients must be fully apprised of these facts and have the goals carefully explained. We cannot merely treat the bladder or the symptom complex but must treat the patient as a whole.

The objective of cystoplasty is bladder enlargement as well as the replacement of the major portion of the diseased bladder with healthy, well-vascularized bowel. In essence, the treatment goal is to convert a high-pressure, non-compliant, small capacity bladder to a low-pressure, compliant, capacious reservoir that will improve or relieve the symptoms of pain and irritability. The pain associated with interstitial cystitis, although not always completely abolished by augmentation, should occur at a higher capacity, thus providing symptomatic relief (George et al. 1978). It is fundamental to ablate most of the bladder wall including a large amount of the nerve supply. The elimination of pain by segmental cystectomy and augmentation cystoplasty is unpredictable; although pain related strictly to bladder filling will probably be abolished or improved, the dyspareunia, urethral burning, and constant pelvic pain will probably not be relieved.

Indications and Patient Selection

Augmentation cystoplasty with supra-trigonal cystectomy is a potential surgical solution to the patient with limited functional bladder capacity and chronic intractable symptoms which have failed to respond to conservative means. Appropriate patient selection is crucial; candidates should have severe frequency, markedly decreased functional capacity, and intractable pain related to filling (Webster and Galloway 1987). Although those with severely reduced capacity under anesthesia will benefit most, those with limited functional capacity but a respectable capacity under anesthesia may also benefit, since the functional capacity is what is responsible for the symptoms.

At the most extreme end of the spectrum of interstitial cystitis, three patterns of pain emerge. There is either a predominance of pain on filling, constant pain independent of the volume status, or a mixed pattern. It appears that the patient with pain on filling but relieved by emptying will be most responsive to augmentation cystoplasty, while the patient with constant pain unrelated to filling or emptying will be most likely to respond to cystectomy. The patient with a mixed pattern is more problematic.

Historical Perspective

Augmentation cystoplasty is not a new procedure, nor has its use been limited to patients with end-stage interstitial cystitis. It has been utilized for contracted bladders secondary to tuberculosis, chemical cystitis, radiation cystitis, and neurogenic impairment. In 1888, Tizzoni and Foggi (Novick et al. 1977) performed a canine ileocystoplasty. This was followed by a human ileocystoplasty performed by Mikuliciz (Kay and Straffon 1986) the following year, and in 1912 Lemoine performed a colocystoplasty. In an attempt to augment the bladder, synthetic materials have been used, but these have been fraught with problems including graft contracture, calculi, infections, fistulas, and metaplastic bone formation. In 1917 Neuhoff (Neuhoff 1917) described the use of a free fascial graft to augment the bladder. Currently, there is abundant ongoing research on synthetic and artificial bladder materials, but until these become clinically useful, bowel will remain the material of choice for augmentation.

Principles and Caveats

Basic principles of augmentation and supra-trigonal cystectomy must be strictly adhered to for optimal results. An adequate amount of bladder must be resected to remove as much of the diseased tissue as possible as well as to prevent detrusor contractions of sufficient magnitude as to allow the cystoplastic segment to function as a large capacity diverticulum. If the diseased bladder is insufficiently resected, the residual tissue may be responsible for producing frequency and sensory urgency despite achievement of an adequate bladder capacity by augmentation (Turner-Warwick and Ashkan 1967).

Generally, the resection margin should be 1 cm above the trigone in an effort not to destroy the ureteral anti-reflux mechanism. Care must be taken to preserve the vascular supply to the trigone, the inferior vesical pedicle which crosses the distal ureters. The bowel segment must be detubularized to modify its contractility. Transecting the circular fibers of the bowel segment will result in improved compliance as compared with the intact loop. The bowel segment must be of sufficient size to allow for the creation of a capacious reservoir and must be carefully mobilized so that it has an adequate blood supply with its mesentery on no tension. The bowel–bladder anastamosis should be wide and stricture free. Stress urinary incontinence must be avoided by bladder neck suspension prior to completing the operation in patients with poor support of the anterior vaginal wall.

Choice of Bowel Segment

The choice of bowel segment has ranged from stomach to sigmoid. Although there are certain inherent advantages and disadvantages to the use of any particular segment, as long as the basic principles and caveats are adhered to, there should not be much difference in results, as reported in a critical review by Smith et al. (1977). Certainly the age of the patient, variation of mesenteric length and mobility, concomitant bowel disease such as diverticulosis, anatomic variations, intra-operative circumstances, and the surgeon's preference will all influence the choice of the segment.

Kay (Kay and Straffon 1986) has succinctly summarized advantages and disadvantages of particular segments. Ileum generally has a long mesentery and is easy to work with although it has a thin wall and will require more length to enlarge a bladder to the extent that can be done with colon. Colon has a large lumen, long mesentery, muscular wall and ureteral reimplants can be performed readily. Sigmoid is advantageous because of its close proximity to the bladder, but secretes copious amounts of mucus, is associated with a higher infection rate, and often coexistent pathology such as diverticular disease is present. An advantage of the ileo-cecal segment becomes evident when there is a need to reimplant the ureters into the ileal component. Turner-Warwick (Turner-Warwick and Ashkan 1967) prefers the cecum since it is easily mobilized, the ileo-colic vasculature is constant and is easily mobilized, rarely is there coexistent cecal pathology, and the ileo-colonic reanastamosis is well away from the cystoplasty, minimizing the chance of a fistula.

At the UCLA Medical Center, our preference is for the ileo-cecal segment because of the advantages documented previously. The use of the ileo-colic segment for augmentation was first described in 1965 by Gil-Vernet (Gil-Vernet 1965) who conceived this segment as a "surgical unit", both anatomic and functional, creating an ideal substitute for both the ureter and the bladder. He reported that this segment provided the advantages of ileocystoplasty and colocystoplasty but none of the disadvantages and superior long-term results.

Our Technique

The abdomen is incised in the midline and the peritoneal cavity entered. The umbilical attachment to the bladder is clamped, divided, and ligated. The dome of the bladder is freed from peritoneal and peri-vesical attachments, and the dissection is carried on to the bladder base. Supra-trigonal cystectomy is then performed using electrocautery to circumferentially excise the bladder approximately one centimeter above the trigone. It is helpful to intubate the ureters with ureteral catheters prior to completing the posterior excision line.

Wide mobilization of the ascending colon, hepatic flexure, and distal ileum is obtained. Transillumination is performed to identify the ileo-colic vascular pedicle, and the proximal and distal mesenteric incisions are made; the vessels are ligated individually. The distal ileum is transected using the GIA stapling device, applying a double row of staples to the proximal and distal ileum. The right colon is transected in a similar fashion. Individual 3-0 silk sutures are applied at the anti-mesenteric borders of the bowel segments and both ends are approximated. A small opening of the anti-mesenteric border of the ileum is made and dilated using fine forceps. One arm of the GIA stapler is inserted. A similar opening of the anti-mesenteric border of the ascending colon is created and the second arm of the GIA stapler is introduced. A side to side double-barrel anastamosis of the proximal ileum and the ascending colon is performed by firing the stapling device. Alice clamps are applied to the bowel edge. The anastamosis is completed using a TA-55 automatic stapler. The patency of the anastamosis is checked by digital examination and the mesenteric trap is closed.

The meso-appendix is isolated, clamped, divided, and ligated. The staple line of the ascending colon is identified and excised. The bowel is irrigated with dilute Betadine solution. The staples in the distal ileum are isolated using a running 3-0 absorbable suture. The cecum is detubularized by incising along the anti-mesenteric tenia using electrocautery for exquisite hemostasis. At mid-distance a 2-0 Vicryl suture is applied to the inferior margin of the cecum. The incision is continued to the base of the appendix and appendectomy is performed.

The cecal-bladder anastamosis is then performed using a continuous one-layer 2-0 Vicryl suture. Several runs of suture are used, starting with the previously placed mid-cecal suture, which is used to secure the middle portion of the inferior wall of the cecum to the middle portion of the posterior wall of the bladder. After completion of the posterior anastamosis, the lateral and anterior anastamosis is completed. A 24 Fr Foley catheter is inserted through a stab wound in the bowel to function as a suprapubic tube. An indwelling urethral Foley catheter is placed as well. Bladder irrigation is done to demonstrate leaks which are secured with suture.

The cecal segment is anchored to the posterior peritoneum above the psoas margin. Two 1-inch Penrose drains are inserted through a stab wound, one placed in the retropubic space and the other in the retrovesical space. The abdominal is closed in layers after thorough irrigation of the abdomen cavity.

The suprapubic and urethral catheters are left indwelling for ten days, and are removed only after a cystogram demonstrates the absence of extravasation.

Series Review

In 1966 Giertz reported 13 patients with a cardinal symptom of pain who failed conservative therapy and underwent subtotal cystectomy and intestinal bladder substitute. This resulted in diminution in pain and increase in capacity in all patients although frequency and nocturia persisted. The results were perceived as excellent in 8, fair in 4, and failure in 1.

In 1970 Koss et al. reported the long-term follow-up of 185 cystoplasties; however, only 3 were done for interstitial cystitis. Colonic bladders seemed to have better functional results than ileal bladders, and results were best for contracted bladders.

In 1974 Futter and Collins urodynamically concluded that success and failure can be clearly differentiated on cystometrogram. All patients with good results had cystometrograms indistinguishable from normal, good capacity, minimal post-void residual, and the ability to suppress the desire to void.

In 1977 Seddon et al. reported the results of 9 cystoplasties in which sigmoid was predominantly used. They reported 7 cures and 2 failures, and interestingly noted the post-operative presence of vesico-ureteral reflux in most patients. Also in 1977 Bruce et al. reported satisfactory relief after cystoplasty in 8 patients with intolerable frequency and painful voiding with an average follow-up of 3 years. Smith et al. (1977) reported 30 augmentations with 68% good–excellent results and 32% failures. They concluded that the detubularized patch was clearly preferable to the tubularized segment and that the choice of bowel segment did not influence the results.

In 1978 George et al. reviewed the late urodynamic results of 19 cystoplasties,

3 of which were done for interstitial cystitis. They concluded that an overall improvement in pain and irritative symptoms occurred, and objectively documented a delay in first desire to void, a decrease in voiding pressure, an increase in capacity, and an increase in post-void residual. Shirley and Mirelman (Shirley and Mirelman 1978) reported mostly good to excellent results in 26 patients after augmentation for interstitial cystitis.

In 1979 Dounis and Gow reported the results of 59 augmentations, 7 of which were done for interstitial cystitis. The interstitial cystitis patients were all treated with cecocystoplasty; all did well with marked symptomatic improvement and a noteworthy reduction in pain and frequency. They also concluded that good results occur regardless of choice of bowel segment. A bladder neck resection or incision was used in all males older than 45 years.

In 1980 Freiha et al. reported 19 patients with intractable interstitial cystitis treated with various open surgical procedures. One patient underwent a segmental resection which only provided temporary relief. Four underwent cystectomy and diversion while 3 underwent diversion alone. Of this diverted group, 6 had permanent relief, 1 committed suicide, and 2 of the 3 unremoved bladders developed pyocystitis. Five patients underwent cystolysis and 6 underwent supra-trigonal cystectomy with cecocystoplasty. Four had lasting relief, but 2 ultimately underwent cystectomy and diversion. At the UCLA Medical Center, 325 patients underwent augmentation cystoplasty in the period 1976-1985. Cystoplasty was done for purposes of augmentation, bypass, undiversion, and substitution. Most of the augmentations were done for neurogenic bladders with small functional capacity.

Ideally, when analyzing the results of surgical therapy for interstitial cystitis, changes in each of the following parameters should be assessed individually:

1. Frequency and urgency
2. Dyspareunia
3. Dysuria
4. Pain on filling
5. Constant pelvic pain
6. Psychosocial dysfunction

Unfortunately, there are no studies which have defined improvements in these terms, and it becomes a very difficult task to compare results in the literature when there exists no uniformity even in defining the symptom complex that we seek to improve through surgical intervention.

Risks and Complications

Although augmentation has generally proved effective in the treatment of refractory interstitial cystitis, it must be understood that this is a major surgical procedure not without complication or risk. The surgeon performing this procedure must be committed to long-term follow-up. Retrospective reviews have indicated the need for more than one operation in up to 30% of patients, and the need for subsequent diversion in up to 25% (Kay and Straffon 1986).

Chronic renal insufficiency defined as a creatinine clearance less than 40 ml/min is a relative contraindication to augmentation because of the risk of absorption of urinary substrates from the absorptive surface of the cystoplastic segment with the potential for metabolic and electrolyte abnormalities, specifically hyperchloremic, hypokalemic metabolic acidosis.

Any general surgical complication inherent to bowel surgery can occur, including ileus, bowel obstruction, anastamotic leak, hernias, pelvic abscess, etc. Bladder problems such as urinary fistula, mucus obstruction, calculi, anastamotic stenosis, chronic urinary infection, and new onset of reflux (Bruce et al. 1977; Shirley and Mirelman 1978), presumably on the basis of intramural damage, can all occur. In the UCLA series of 325 augmentations, early complications included 2 bowel fistulas, 5 cases of prolonged ileus, and 1 bowel infarct. Late complications included symptomatic urinary infections in 15%, hour-glass anastamotic narrowing in 5 cases, mucus plugging requiring irrigation in 3%, and bladder calculi in 3%. McGuire et al. (1973) reported an interesting complication of cystoplasty in which a patient did well for 16 months after which time the symptoms recurred and cystoscopy and biopsy demonstrated an inflammatory infiltrate with increased vascularity and fibrosis consistent with interstitial cystitis in the cystoplastic segment. After intra-vesical steroid treatment, the symptoms abated and the biopsy normalized.

Turner-Warwick (1979) reported that the replacement of effective detrusor contraction by ineffective peristaltic evacuation of detubularized bowel will often result in a voiding imbalance which may require an adjustment of outflow resistance. Bowel peristalsis is autonomically mediated and not under voluntary control, is stimulated by distension, and activity tends to fade during emptying. An augmentation cystoplasty characteristically shows uninhibitable peristaltic contractions between voiding, but these are unsustained during voiding, leaving a residual. Most patients learn to complete voiding, but these are unsustained during voiding, leaving a residual. Most patients learn to complete voiding by abdominal straining. A simple solution to the problem of voiding dysfunction is self-catheterization. In the UCLA experience with augmentation cystoplasty, self-catheterization has been needed in almost 30% of the non-neurogenic group.

Fall and Nilsson (1982) take a conservative attitude towards cystoplasty, reserving it only for use when the bladder capacity is less than 150 ml and disabling pain is present. In a series of 12 patients, they reported 7 with good results and 5 with no improvement. They demonstrated an alarming incidence of marked sensory urgency after cystoplasty. In the clinical situation of pronounced urethral pain, and/or local lesions within or close to the trigone, they emphasize the possible need for trigonal resection. Kay and Straffon (1986) suggested that symptoms remaining after augmentation may be due to hyper-excitable afferent impulses from the trigone, contributed to by inflammatory involvement of the trigonal nerve supply. He concluded that not all symptoms are due to small bladder capacity and neither simple augmentation nor excision of the majority of the bladder will be successful in all patients.

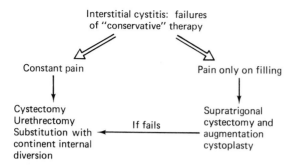

Fig. 22.1. Surgical therapy of interstitial cystitis.

Cystectomy and Total Bladder Substitution

It is for the population of interstitial cystitis patients with chronic disabling bladder pain independent of filling status and patients unimproved after augmentation that the most radical of all treatments, total cystectomy, is reserved (Fig. 22.1). A simple urinary diversion without cystectomy is a viable alternative for the high-risk elderly patient. Many forms of diversion have been employed, with the ileal conduit most commonly utilized. Other forms of continent diversion including the Koch pouch, the Mainz pouch, etc., have come into vogue and have been used with increasing frequency. At UCLA Medical Center we have been using total cystectomy and urethrectomy with reconstruction of the neo-urethra using intussuscepted ileocecal valve, substitution of the bladder using the ileocecal segment patched onto an additional ileal segment and reimplantation of both ureters into the cecum.

Surgical Technique

With the patient in the frog leg position, a total cystectomy and urethrectomy is performed. Prior to transection, holding sutures of 2-0 Vicryl are placed on the urethral cuff. A sponge stick in the vagina facilitates dissection of the bladder and urethra from anterior vaginal wall. The ureters are transected adjacent to the bladder and the lateral attachments of the vagina and endopelvic fascia are dissected. For patients with poor support of the anterior vaginal wall, a Burch bladder neck suspension is performed using No. 1 Vicryl to suspend the lateral vaginal wall to Cooper's ligament. These sutures will provide support to the neourethra and will be tied only after completion of the anastamosis. The levators and pubocervical Gascia are approximated behind the uretha to reconstitute the pelvic floor.

The ileocecal segment is isolated in standard fashion as previously described; 20 cm of ascending colon and 40 cm of distal ileum are used. A side to side double-barrel anastamosis of the ascending colon and distal ileum is performed with the automatic stapling device and the mesenteric trap is closed. At a distance of 15 cm from the ileocecal valve the GIA stapler is applied, separating two bowel segments; the ileocecal segment that will be used for creation of the neourethra, bladder base and ureteric reimplantation, and a second segment of 25 cm of ileum that will be used as a patch for augmentation only. The cecum is opened along its antimesenteric tenia to the level of the appendix which is removed in continuity, thereby creating a patch of cecum. The distal 6 cm of distal ileum is cleaned of its mesentery and the terminal ileum is intussuscepted into the cecum using three rows of S-GIA staples. One row of staples is applied to the nipple and the wall of the cecum for fixation. After a 32 Fr catheter is placed in the intussuscepted ileum, a ring of Dexon mesh is applied and interrupted 3-0 Prolene sutures are used to incorporate ileal wall, Dexon mesh, and cecal wall. After intussusception, the afferent limb of the ileum is 2–3 cm long. The ileal anastamosis to the urethral stump is performed with interrupted sutures of 2-0 Vicryl. A 32 Fr Medina catheter is placed through the anastamosis and is secured to the anterior abdominal wall by placing a Nylon suture through the catheter tip; this will prevent inadvertent catheter displacement.

The ureters are reimplanted into the cecum using a submucosal anti-refluxing tunnel, and double pigtail catheters are placed. The isolated ileal segment is folded in U-shaped fashion, opened on its anti-mesenteric border, fashioned as a pouch, and anastamosed to the opened cecal segment with a 2-0 Vicryl running suture. A 22 Fr Foley catheter is placed through the cecal wall to function as a suprapubic tube. The vaginal suspension sutures are tied and the anterior aspect of the neo-bladder is secured to the posterior aspect of the anterior abdominal wall to prevent kinking and facilitate self-catheterization. The abdomen is irrigated after irrigation of the neo-bladder demonstrates a water-tight anastamosis. Peri-vesical Penrose drains are placed and the abdomen is closed in standard fashion.

Results and Complications

This technique has been used on eight patients during the past 4-year period and has required a mean operative time of four hours and a mean hospital stay of 9 days. Average follow-up is 18 months. Four patients remain continent on self-catheterization and all have documented capacious low-pressure, compliant, non-refluxing neo-bladders and normal upper tracts. Several patients required further surgery including one requiring a revision of the nipple, one with hematuria who required endoscopic removal of an exposed staple, two patients who required excision of their native distal urethral stump for persistent pain due to interstitial cystitis, and one patient who required a uterine suspension for uterine prolapse. Four patients ultimately required cystectomy of the continent pouch because of continuous pain and/or infection. These 4 were treated with ileal conduit diversion, rendering 3 pain free, but 1 had continued pain.

Our substitute satisfies the criteria of a low pressure, compliant, capacious reservoir which can be emptied efficiently, maintains continence, and preserves upper tract function by avoiding reflux and obstruction. However, long-term follow-up has documented that urinary infections and pain are significant problems in half the patients treated with substitution. For the carefully selected patient, this form of continent internal urinary diversion may offer promise for creating a functional bladder substitute without an external stoma.

References

Borque JP (1951) Surgical management of the painful bladder. J Urol 65:25

Bruce P, Buckham C, Carden A, Salvaris M (1977) The surgical treatment of chronic interstitial cystitis. Med J Aust 1:581–582

Bumpus HC (1930) Interstitial cystitis; its treatment by over distension of the bladder. Med Clin North Am 13:1495

Dounis A, Gow JG (1979) Bladder augmentation: a long-term review. Br J Urol 51:264–268

Dunn M, Ramsden PD, Roberts JBM, Smith JC, Smith PJP (1977) Interstitial cystitis, treatment by prolonged bladder distention. Br J Urol 49:641–645

Ewing R, Bultitude MI, Shuttleworth KED (1982) Subtrigonal phenol injection for urge incontinence secondary to detrusor instability. Br J Urol 54:689–692

Fall M (1985) Management of chronic interstitial cystitis: transcutaneous electrical nerve stimulation and transurethral resection. J Urol 133:774–778

Fall M, Nilsson S (1982) Volume augmentation cystoplasty and persistent urgency. Scand J Urol Nephrol 16:125–128

Freiha F, Stamey T (1980) Cystolysis: a procedure for the selective denervation of the bladder. J Urol 123:360–363

Freiha F, Faysal M, Stamey T (1980) The surgical treatment of intractable interstitial cystitis. J Urol 123:632–634

Futter NG, Collins WE (1974) Intestinal cystoplasty: long-term functional results. Urology 3:434

George N, Dunn M, Dounis A, Abrams P, Smith P (1978) The late symptomatic and functional results of enterocystoplasty. Br J Urol 50:517–520

Giertz G (1966) Interstitial cystitis: 13 patients treated operatively with intestinal bladder substitutes. Acta Chir Scand 132:436

Gil-Vernet J (1965) The ileo-colic segment in urologic surgery. J Urol 98:418–426

Greenberg E, Barnes R, Stewart S, Furnish T (1974) Transurethral resection of Hunner's ulcers. J Urol 111:764–766

Hanash KA, Pool TL (1969) Interstitial cystitis in men. J Urol 102:427–430

Hanno PM, Wein AJ (1987) Interstitial cystitis. AUA Update Series, vol. 6, lessons 9–10

Hunner CH (1918) Elusive ulcer of the bladder. Am J Obstet 78:374

Kay R, Straffon R (1986) Augmentation cystoplasty. Urol Clin North Am 13:295–305

Koss R, Bitker M, Camey M, Chatelain C, Lassau JP (1970) Indications and early and late results of intestinal cystoplasty: a review. J Urol 103:53–63

Lapides J (1975) Observations on interstitial cystitis. Urology 5:610–611

Leach GE, Raz S (1983) Interstitial cystitis. In: Raz S (ed) Female urology. Saunders, Philadelphia, pp 351–356

McGuire EJ, Lytton B, Cornog Jr JL (1973) Interstitial cystitis following colocystoplasty. Urology 1:28–29

Messing EM (1986) Interstitial cystitis and related syndromes. In: Walsh PC, Gittes RF, Perlmutter AD, Stamey TA (eds) Campbell's urology, 5th edition. Saunders, Philadelphia, pp 1070–1092

Messing EM, Stamey TA (1978) Interstitial cystitis: Early diagnosis, pathology, and treatment. Urology 12:381–392

Neuhoff H (1917) Fascia transplantation into visceral defect. Surg Gynecol Obstet 24:383

Novick AC, Straffon RA, Banowsky LH et al. (1977) Experimental bladder substitution using biodegradable graft of natural tissue. Urology 10:118-127

Oravisto KJ (1975) Epidemiology of interstitial cystitis. Ann Chir Gynaecol Fenn 64:75–77

Pool TL (1967) Interstitial cystitis: clinical considerations and treatment. Clin Obstet Gynecol 10:185–191

Seddon J, Best L, Bruce A (1977) Intestinocystoplasty in the treatment of interstitial cystitis. Urology 5:431–435

Shanberg AM, Baghdassarian R, Tansey LA (1985) Treatment of interstitial cystitis with the neodymium-yag laser. J Urol 134:885–888

Shirley SW, Mirelman S (1978) Experience with colocystoplasties, cecocystoplasties, and ileocystoplasties in urologic surgery: 40 patients. J Urol 120:165–168

Smith RB, VanCangh P, Skinner DG, Kaufman JJ, Goodwin WE (1977) Augmentation enterocystoplasty: a critical review. J Urol 118:35–39

Torrens M, Hald T (1979) Bladder denervation procedures. Urol Clin North Am 6:283–293

Turner-Warwick RT (1979) Cystoplasty. Urol Clin North Am 1:259–264

Turner-Warwick RT, Ashkan MH (1967) The functional results of partial, subtotal, and total cystoplasty with special reference to ureterocecocystoplasty, selective sphincterotomy, and cystocystoplasty. Br J Urol 39:3–12

Webster CD, Galloway N (1987) Surgical treatment of interstitial cystitis: indications, techniques, and results. Urology Suppl 29:34–39

Worth PHL (1980) The treatment of interstitial cystitis by cystolysis with observations on cystoplasty. A review after seven years. Br J Urol 52:232

Worth P, Turner-Warwick RT (1973) The treatment of interstitial cystitis by cystolysis with observations on cystoplasty. Br J Urol 45:65–71

Editorial Comment

Substitution Cystoplasty in the Management of Interstitial Cystitis

G. D. Webster

There is no panacea in the treatment of interstitial cystitis. Supratrigonal cystectomy and substitution cystoplasty should be reserved for those few patients for whom all other conservative remedies have failed and whose disabilities are such that supravesical urinary diversion might otherwise be considered. Such strict selection criteria are necessary in view of the enigmatic nature of the disease, the subjective nature of symptoms, and the fact that this is a relatively major operative procedure for a condition which might otherwise offer little risk to health or life.

It has been suggested that candidates for cystoplasty should be patients with longstanding intractable symptoms in whom the true bladder capacity under anesthesia is markedly reduced. This argument has been supported mainly by anecdotal evidence. However, it was also the conclusion of this author's own study of 19 cases undergoing cystoplasty in whom preoperative capacities under anesthesia ranged from 100 to 550 ml (mean 265 ml) (Webster and Maggio 1988). The 12 patients who experienced excellent relief of symptoms had bladder capacities between 100 and 350 ml (mean 190 ml) whilst a group of 4 women who experienced only partial relief of symptoms had preoperative capacities of 300 to 550 ml (mean 450 ml). The remaining 3 patients who failed to improve at all after cystoplasty, and who ultimately underwent urinary diversion, similarly had larger capacities but in addition had voiding problems requiring intermittent self-catheterization. This combination of residual bladder/urethral hypersensitivity symptoms and the need to self-catheterize is a very emotive situation and is poorly tolerated by these already distraught patients.

Figure E.1 demonstrates our surgical technique. Postoperatively the patient is managed with a suprapubic and urethral Foley catheter, the Foley being removed on the 7th day and the suprapubic once a successful voiding trial has been completed, which is usually at approximately the 14th to 18th postoperative days. In this author's series of 9 patients, 5 were unable to void efficiently after cystoplasty. However, of these, 4 had contributing reasons (prior bilateral S3 denervation in two, simultaneously performed cystourethropexy which "unbalanced" the system in 1 and total cystectomy down to the bladder neck in 1) and in only one case was retention unexpected. Nonetheless, it is important that patients being considered for this management understand the risk and accept the prospect of self-catheterization.

It is our impression that paramount to success is the aggressive removal of diseased bladder and the construction of a capacious reservoir. Only a 1 cm rim

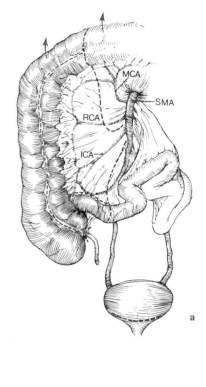

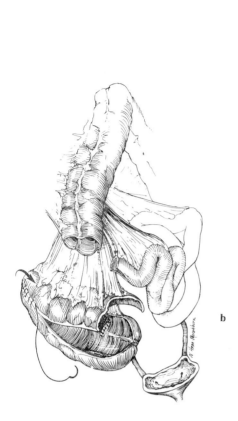

b

a

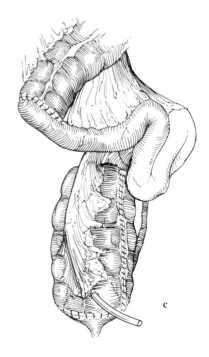

c

Fig. E.1a–c. a Following supratrigonal bladder resection, a cystoplasty of adequate capacity will require use of the entire right colon almost as far as the middle colic artery (MCA). The right colic artery (RCA) may be sacrificed for the entire segment will remain viable on the ileocecal artery (ICA) by way of the marginal artery. A small terminal segment of ileum and appendix may be discarded. **b** Ileotransverse reanastomosis is accomplished. The isolated segment of right colon is detubularized and remodeled by folding as shown. Aggressive supratrigonal bladder resection is accomplished leaving a 1 cm rim above the bladder neck and interureteric ridge, and a slightly larger rim over the intramural ureter. **c** Colovesical anastomosis is completed. Both suprapubic and urethral catheter drainage are necessary in the immediate postoperative period. Ideally the system is wrapped in an omental pedicle to preserve functional mobility (not shown).

of bladder should be left above the trigone and bladder neck, a slightly more generous allowance being allowed over the intramural ureters, so as to avoid later reflux. We have not seen the typical endoscopic features of interstitial cystitis on the trigone (perhaps because this area is rather indistensible). For this reason subtrigonal resection of the bladder was never performed as a primary procedure in our patients and it is also certainly true that sparing the trigone preserves some important bladder sensation (and function) necessary to maintain voiding ability.

Bowel selection for cystoplasty is largely a matter of personal preference, and whilst functional differences do exist between sigmoid, right colon and ileum, detubularization and remodeling techniques will largely ablate any undesirable high-pressure overactivity. It has been this author's preference to use the right colon, basing the segment on the ileocolic pedicle. It produces a capacious reservoir and it easily approximates the bladder remnant.

It is certainly this author's impression that for a small select group of patients this is appropriate management, the excellent outcome in 63% seeming to justify the approach. The alternative would be for patients to continue to live with intractable symptoms or to undergo a urinary diversion. Late failures seem uncommon, and it is likely that our results do reflect a long-term success. It is hoped that with the passage of time, selection criteria will become better established. However, it seems more likely that ultimately the identification of the true etiology of this condition will lead to the establishment of more logical non-operative intervention.

Reference

Webster GD, Maggio MI (1989) The management of chronic interstitial cystitis by substitution cystoplasty. J Urol 141:287–291

Addendum. Summary of the 1989 AUA Podium Section on Genitourinary Infection: Interstitial Cystitis

Prepared by K. E. Whitmore

The first AUA podium session devoted entirely to the subject of interstitial cystitis (moderators: C. L . Parsons and T. J. Rohner) provided interesting and informative reviews on histology, etiology (infections, biochemical, immunologic), urinary constituents (glycosaminoglycans), surface active agents (DMSO, oxycholorosene) and treatment (amitriptyline).

Histology of Interstitial Cystitis

W. L. Lynes, S. Flynn, L. D. Shortliffe and T. A. Stamey (Upland, California)

Histological parameters among control and IC patients were studied. IC patients were divided into two groups based on bladder capacity under anesthesia (normal >400 ml), and the presence or absence of pyuria. IC patients with small bladder capacities and/or pyuria, when compared to controls or IC patients with normal bladder capacities and no pyuria, had significant epithelial loss, ulceration, and greater than Grade II submucosal inflammation. This group of patients also responded better to therapy than did normal capacity, no pyuria patients. The authors suggested that biopsies may be helpful in the diagnosis of IC only if a small bladder capacity or pyuria is present.

Silver Staining of Mucosal Biopsy Specimens in Chronic Interstitial Cystitis: Is There a Bacterial Etiology?

S. W. Siegel, B. Guz and P. Suit (Cleveland, Ohio)

The bacterium *Campylobacter pylori* is readily detected histologically by the Dieterle silver stain, and has been identified as a likely specific cause of gastrointestinal inflammatory disorders. Fourteen female patients with chronic IC, who met the NIDDK criteria for diagnosis had negative silver stains for *Campylobacter pylori* on bladder biopsy specimens when compared with positive controls, (gastric mucosal biopsy specimens positive for *Campylobacter pylori* on silver staining). It was suggested that these results added to the evidence that IC does not have a bacterial etiology.

The Evidence for Occult Bacterial Infections as a Cause of Interstitial Cystitis

W. L. Lynes, R. G. Sellers and L. D. Shortliffe (Stanford, California)

Twelve healthy subjects and 12 IC patients were studied to determine whether routine or fastidious organisms, or an immunologic reaction could be an etiologic factor in IC. Routine C and S was negative in all patients. There was no significant difference between healthy and IC patients in antibody titers to routine Gram positive (*Staphylococcus, Streptococcus*) organisms or to IgA and IgG antibodies, by ELISA assay, in serum and concentrated morning urine specimens. In addition, serum antibody titers to *Chlamydia* and *Ureaplasma urealyticum* by ELISA assay, showed no significant difference. The authors concluded that there was no evidence of recent or remote Gram negative or positive infections in the patients with IC, and the lack of increased total urinary IgA or IgG, may make infection by an untested organism, antibiotic reaction, or immunogenic substance unlikely as an etiologic factor for IC.

Increased Transvesical Small Molecule Movement in Patients with Interstitial Cystitis

J. D. Lilly and C. L. Parsons (San Diego, California)

This study was based on a previous report in 27 normal volunteers which showed that the small molecule urea traversed the bladder wall; this movement increased significantly following the intravesical instillation of protamine sulfate, (which produced irritable bladder symptoms), with levels returning to near normal following the instillation of heparin sulfate. The transvesical movement of urea was studied in 11 patients with IC, 2 in remission and 9 symptomatic. Five of the 9 symptomatic IC patients who tolerated urea instillation had greater movement of urea out of the bladder than the 2 IC patients in remission and the previous normal volunteers. This permeability was reversed with the instillation of heparin sulfate. The authors concluded that the epithelium in IC patients is "leaky" to small molecules. In addition, protamine sulfate appears to produce small molecule movement and irritative bladder symptoms, and is thought to inactivate the glycosaminoglycan layer, which can be replaced with exogenous heparin.

Characterization of Cellular Immunity in Interstitial Cystitis

J. P MacDermott, A. R. Stone, C. H. Miller and N. Levy (Sacramento, California)

Monoclonal antibodies to lymphocyte subsets, (pan-B, pan-T, helper/inducer T, suppressor/cytotoxic T, and monocyte/macrophage) were used to study the phenotyping of the inflammatory cells present in the bladder wall in IC patients. Most of the bladder wall lymphocytes in IC patients were subset helper/inducer T cells whose serum lymphocyte subsets were completely normal. The significance of these findings, which are at variance with previous results showing normal lymphocytes in the urinary tract, remains to be determined.

Tamm-Horsfall Protein Antibody in Interstitial Cystitis

J. P. Dilworth, D. E. Neal, Jr. and M. B. Kaack (New Orleans, Louisiana)

Eight patients with clinical (for more than one year), cystoscopic, and histologic IC (chronic inflammation and mast cells) were studied to determine the absorption of Tamm-Horsfall protein (THP – previously identified in the superficial urothelium of IC patients as evidence of abnormal urothelial permeability) through the urothelium. IC patients had a significantly greater serum anti-THP antibody (IgG by ELISA assay with mean 2750) as compared to controls (mean 114), indicating humoral response to THP and suggesting that the normal urothelial barrier to absorption of substances in urine is lost in IC. The authors concluded that measurement of serum THP antibody may prove to be useful as a noninvasive diagnostic test in patients with IC.

Increased Urinary Glycosaminoglycan Excretion after Bladder Distension in Interstitial Cystitis Patients

R. E. Hurst, J. B. Roy and J. L. Young (Oklahoma City, Oklahoma)

This study was done to determine if bladder overdistention and relief of pain and urgency symptoms were associated with decreased urinary GAG values. Four IC patients had a significant increase in urinary GAG excretion following overdistension, when compared with pre-treatment values, that persisted up to 30 days after treatment. The results were interpreted to mean that the relief afforded by bladder distension is accompanied by an increase in urinary GAG excretion, and may stimulate growth of urothelium or increased surface GAG biosynthesis.

Effects of Intravesical DMSO

A. Freedman, R. M. Levin, K. E. Whitmore and A. J. Wein (Philadelphia, Pennsylvania)

This study was designed to evaluate the effects of intravesical instillation of DMSO on bladder physiology and function. Instillation of 50% DMSO into male White New Zealand rabbits produced a marked decrease in bladder capacity and diminished response to field stimulation (peak pressure and percent emptying). This effect decreased with time but never approached initial values. The authors concluded that intravesical DMSO instillation appears to have a significant negative effect on bladder function.

Effectiveness of Oxychlorosene (Chlorpactin[tm]) in Interstitial Cystitis

T. J. Rohner (Hershey, Pennsylvania)

Thirty-seven patients with clinical, cystoscopic, and histologic IC who benefited from hydraulic dilation and instillation of 0.4% oxychlorosene under anesthesia, were studied. Fourteen patients without IC derived no relief from hydraulic dilation or oxychlorosene instillation. Of the 37 (59%) IC patients who benefited from initial hydraulic dilation and instillation, 6 (16%) required no further therapy after 1–9 years of follow-up; and 16 (43%) benefited from repeated instillations of 0.2% oxychlorosene at 3 to 18 month intervals. This form of therapy proved efficacious with results equalling or bettering other forms of bladder instillation therapy for IC.

Amitriptyline in the Treatment of Interstitial Cystitis

P. M. Hanno (Philadelphia, Pennsylvania)

Forty-three female IC patients, (mean age 42 years, average 47 months of symptoms, bladder capacity under anesthesia 300–1300 mL, and no Hunner's ulcers), who were refractory to hydrodistension of the bladder under anesthesia and DMSO bladder instillations, were treated with amitriptyline on an incremental dosing schedule (35 mg, 50 mg, 75 mg per day). Of the 28 available patients able to tolerate the therapy for at least 3 weeks, 18 had total remissions (mean 14.4 months), 5 dropped out because of side effects, and 5 had no benefit at all. A trial of amitriptyline therapy for IC patients refractory to standard therapy was recommended.

Subject Index